MW01518711

Souper Slim at 70
I lost 25 lbs.

228 Low-Fat
and Low-Sugar Recipes
(64 Soups)

Eileen Tesch

Eileen Tesch

First Printing............................March, 2003

Souper Slim at 70
© 2003 by Eileen Tesch
All rights reserved. No part may be reproduced in
any form, or by any means, electronic or
mechanical, without written permission of the
author, except a reviewer who may use a recipe in
a newspaper or magazine article.

ISBN #0-9671762-9-8

Published by:
HEINS PUBLICATIONS
Rev. William A. Heins
2016 Leonard Ct.
Eau Claire WI 54703-9000
Tel. #'s: 715.874.6677
Toll-free: 800.55HEINS (800.554.3467)

Dedicated to my children

Dennis & Mary
Daughter-in-Law Sandy
Grandchildren
Brian, Laura, Carmen

Inspiration

In the past I ran across this inspirational piece. It has helped me, perhaps it will help you, also.

Accept it as a way of life.

Believe in the psychology of it.

Be patient.

Give plenty of time.

Leave room for error.

Expect things to be different.

Keep a sense of humor.

Keep putting one foot in front of the other.

Have faith in yourself.

Keep the faith and desire to do it and also the strength.

Just be me.

Think Thin.

Introduction

When the scale reached a certain point, I decided, "This is it, I'm going to lose weight."

I started reading and looking for something I could live with. I didn't want to lose weight and end up gaining it back, as I did years ago. Also, I'm not very good at following a prescribed diet for any length of time.

I read a lot of different suggestions, and most of them call for salads everyday, which after a time I lost interest. So, I decided to sometimes put the vegetables or fruit in a soup. In fact, I usually did it this way. Some of the soups can be frozen, so would sometimes freeze a serving or two.

In my readings, suggestions were made of not combining certain foods, so thought why not try it. I usually don't eat animal protein with bread or potatoes. Usually I ate potatoes or bread between meals, or as a snack, or for lunch with a vegetable or vegetable soup.

When I ate out, I would order a protein and a vegetable or salad or vegetable soup, but didn't eat bread or potato with my meal. If something looked good that I'm not eating, I'll take it home in a take-home box and have it the next day.

I ate my protein with a vegetable, cooked or in a

salad or soup.

Also, I had a sandwich with vegetables only, like lettuce, tomatoes, broccoli, asparagus, mushrooms, eggplant, etc. The recipes are in the book.

I got away from snacking on corn chips, etc. At first I allowed myself a few as a treat, but now have cut them out; it's just not worth gaining some weight back.

I didn't take any pills or medication of any kind for reducing. I take a multivitamin/multimineral supplement pill a day.

I allowed myself 100 calories a day treat. Whatever I was hungry for, within reason, otherwise I'm afraid I would fail at losing weight and keeping it off. I do allow myself an occasional treat, but the next day I take it easy.

Oh how many times I said, "If only I could lose 10, 15 or 20 pounds." I finally did it. I've kept the weight off for over two years!

Suggestions

In my recipes I usually use frozen vegetables and fruit. They're just as nutritious and you spend less time preparing the recipes. You can use fresh vegetables and fruits in the recipes if you prefer, especially when they're in season. I've tried to keep the ingredients simple and easy to prepare, also eliminating a lot of the fat and sugar, or cut down on them. Some recipes take a little longer.

Use unsweetened frozen fruit juice concentrate, such as pineapple, apple, grape, orange, etc. Spoon out the desired amount undiluted to fruit soups.

I usually use vegetable broth in my vegetable soups; have also used turkey, beef and chicken broth. Or, make your own. I buy a broth base in a jar and make my broth from that, or you can buy canned broth.

If you don't want herb leaves in your soup or dish, put them in a stainless steel strainer or infuser with a lid, or tie them in a cheese cloth bag, like 1 clove crushed garlic, couple sprigs parsley, black peppercorns, basil, etc. Combine it with your broth or make a broth this way, adding some onions, celery and carrots, etc.

I also used powdered milk a lot, put in a little more of the dry milk than the recipe calls for to the water to get more calcium.

When sautéing onions for a recipe, sauté a couple large onions and freeze the leftover amount in 1/2 cup serving size, or a larger bag laid flat, and can break off amount needed, cutting down on the time for preparing the next recipe.

When having bread, dip it in olive oil sprinkled with dipping herbs. I bought a bread dipping set with mixed herbs.

Have a salad bar, appetizers or relish tray with some of the easy to make relishes, such as red cabbage, green peas, kraut relish, kidney beans, etc.. The recipes are in the book. Have a soup or two, also fruit soup or fruit for dessert, or with bread or a protein.

Having a cookout, just don't eat bread or potato with your meat. Have lots of vegetable and fruit dishes with your meal.

If you work, take along a serving of vegetable or soup and a couple crackers, bun or slice of bread or a protein for your lunch. Take along a fruit or fruit soup for a break, or have some fat-free cottage cheese or 1 ounce low-fat cheese with cut up mixed fruit. When I have a fruit salad, I try to have 3 different colors, like strawberries, blueberries, pineapple chunks or peach slices. I keep the fruit stocked in the freezer; of course, fresh is excellent. Take a short walk 20 minutes or so before you eat, then sit back and relax.

I cut down drastically on saturated fat. When I shop, I look at the nutritional guide. If the saturated fat is higher than 3-4%, I don't buy it. The snack crackers, plain oatmeal cookie and the ginger snaps I buy have 3-4%; they are available. Also, any food or candy that has palm kernel oil or coconut oil in the ingredients, I don't buy it.

I made a menu out for a week. That way I had the ingredients and didn't think, "what am I going to have today," and then have something I shouldn't have eaten. I also kept the menu and filed it. If I had a good week at losing some weight, I might have repeated it or made a notation on it. Also, they're handy for the next time you're planning a menu; just use one of those in the file.

I tried to keep my meals nutritious, eating from all of the food groups.

I have some lower calorie dessert recipes in the book, but while you're losing weight, don't eat any or have a very small piece for your treat.

When you go shopping at a mall, don't park in front of the store you're planning to go to; park at the opposite end of the mall. Also, any store or place you plan on going to.

I tried to walk about 30 minutes, three times a week. Also, I did eat a lot of the soups. I usually had a 3-ounce ground turkey patty, lamb chop, salmon, tuna or other protein with the soup. Sometimes I had a fruit soup for breakfast or as a snack. There's a great variety of soup recipes. Here's hoping you find some to your liking.

The recipes in this book are low fat or no fat, low sugar or no sugar. They are not as rich as most recipes. That's the idea of it, to cut down on rich foods and lose weight.

Good luck!

100 Calorie Treat Suggestions

2 Fig Newtons

2 ginger snaps

3-4 Hershey's Kisses, 1 tablespoon semi-sweet
chocolate chips, or your favorite piece of candy.

16 miniature pretzels

3 baked pretzel rods

1/4 cup oyster crackers

2 graham crackers

1 rice cake with 2 teaspoons peanut butter

1 rice cake with 2 tablespoons fat-free cream cheese,
sprinkled with cinnamon

3-5 dried apricot halves

3-5 prunes

3-5 dates

2-3 dried figs

1/2 cup fat free and sugar free frozen yogurt or ice
cream.

2 cups air popped popcorn

3 tablespoons roasted soy nuts

6 almonds or 6 cashews, 3 walnuts or 10 peanuts
(can use as your fat allowance)

Garnishes

Cut strips of cooked macaroni to make tiny rings.

Chopped fresh chives, mint, parsley, watercress, dill weed, etc., or a sprig of herbs.

Dollop of fat free sour cream or plain yogurt sprinkled with herbs or spices.

Slivered pimento.

Sliced ripe or green olives.

Grated cheese.

Chopped onions.

Lemon, lime, orange slices or wedges.

Croutons.

Thinly sliced sautéed frankfurters or pepperoni.

Lightly sprinkle with paprika, cinnamon, nutmeg, mace, etc.

TABLE OF CONTENTS

Chapter 3 Salads, Relishes, Sauces

Chapter 4 Soups

Chapter 5 Main Dishes

Chapter 6 Meats, Poultry, Fish

Chapter 7 Pasta, Rice

Chapter 8 Sandwiches, Breads

Chapter 9 Vegetables

Chapter 10 Desserts

Recipes

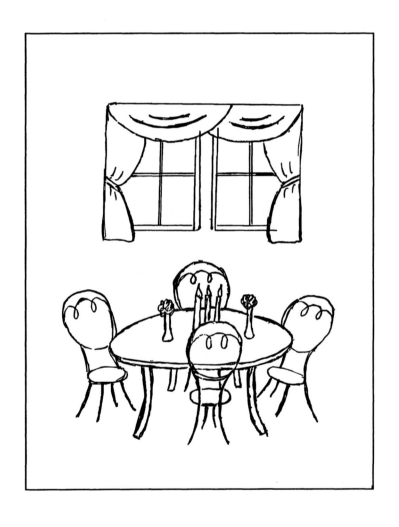

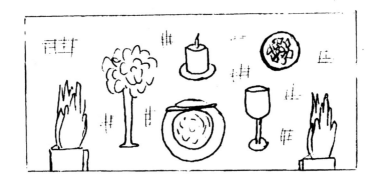

Chapter 1

Appetizers
Dips
Beverages

Spinach Squares

3 eggs
1 cup milk
1 cup flour
½ teaspoon salt
½ teaspoon baking powder
10 oz. frozen spinach, thawed & squeezed
1 cup grated low-fat cheese (Colby, cheddar
     or mozzarella)
¼ cup chopped onions

Preheat oven to 350 degrees. Spray a 9 x 17 inch pan or 9 x 13-inch pan.

Beat eggs, add milk, flour, salt & baking powder & mix well. Stir in spinach, cheese & onions. Spoon into baking pan.

Bake 35 minutes. Remove from oven & let set 45 minutes. Cut into 24 squares.

8-12 Servings.

Vegetable Pizza

8 ounce low-fat crescent rolls
8 ounces fat free cream cheese
½ cup fat free mayonnaise
½ teaspoon dill weed
½ teaspoon mustard
½ teaspoon garlic powder

Lay crescent rolls flat on ungreased cookie sheet. If should separate some, press together. Bake in 350 degree oven for 10-12 minutes. Cool.

Combine cream cheese, mayonnaise, dill weed, mustard & garlic powder. Spread on cooled crust.

Finely chop fresh vegetables. Such as green onion, cauliflower, broccoli, ripe & green olives. Steam broccoli & cauliflower 5 minutes if desired. Put chopped vegetables over mayonnaise mixture. Chill.

Cut into 24 squares.

Homemade Summer Sausage

2 pounds ground round or ground sirloin
½ cup water
1½ teaspoons liquid smoke
½ teaspoon garlic powder
½ teaspoon onion powder
2 tablespoons Morton's quick cure
¼ teaspoon salt

Mix all ingredients together & roll into two rolls. Wrap each roll in aluminum foil. Refrigerate 24 hours.

Poke holes in bottom of rolls. Place on a rack in a baking pan. Bake in a slow oven, 325 degrees for 1¼ hours.

Refrigerate 3 days before using. Cut into thin slices.

Keeps very well in refrigerator.

15 Servings.

Sweet & Sour Meatballs

12 ounce bottle chili sauce
2-8 ounce cans cranberry sauce
1 lemon
1 medium size cabbage
3 pounds ground chuck or ground round
1 teaspoon salt
¼ teaspoon pepper
1 tablespoon soy sauce

Pour the chili sauce & cranberry sauce in large pan on top of stove. Add the juice of the lemon. Cut up the cabbage into small pieces & add to the mixture. Cover & cook slowly for one half hour.

Season the meat with salt, pepper & soy sauce & form into small meatballs. Drop them carefully, unbrowned, into the mixture in the pan, cover & cook slowly for 45 minutes.

When the meatballs are made tiny & served as hors d'oeuvres, will serve 24 people.

Large sized meatballs as a dinner entrée will serve 8-10 people.

Nutritious Bars

1½ cups oatmeal (dry)
3 cups puffed rice cereal
¾ cup whole bran cereal
1 teaspoon cinnamon
½ cup frozen apple juice concentrate
½ cup molasses
½ cup raisins
1/3 cup dried apricots, chopped

Combine cereals and cinnamon in a large bowl, add apple juice concentrate and molasses, mix ingredients. Stir in raisins and apricots, mix well.

Pour into a 9 x 11 inch vegetable sprayed baking pan. Press mixture down firmly.

Bake in 275 degrees oven for 50 – 55 minutes.

Remove from oven, let cool slightly before slicing.

15 Servings.

Onion Bread Squares

8 ounce refrigerated low-fat crescent rolls
2 medium size onions, cut into fourths,
      then sliced
2 tablespoons olive oil
1 egg
8 ounces fat free sour cream
½ teaspoon salt
½ teaspoon dill weed

Put crescent rolls in a 9x12 inch ungreased pan, pressing dough together to cover bottom.

Sauté onions in oil in frying pan until soft. Meanwhile beat egg slightly; blend in sour cream, salt & dill weed.

Spoon softened onions on top of dough. Spoon sour cream mixture over onions.

Bake in 375 degree oven (350 if pan is glass) for 30 minutes or until topping is set.

Cut into 24 squares or wedges, serve warm.

6-8 Servings.

Yogurt Cheese

1-16 ounce container gelatin-free nonfat yogurt

Line strainer with a coffee filter & set over deep bowl. Pour yogurt into coffee filter, cover with plastic wrap & refrigerate 4 hours or overnight. Cheese is ready to eat when it has reduced to 1 cup.

Can add some seasoning to yogurt.

Refrigerate, covered for up to 4 days.

Can be used in dips, dessert & as an alternative to cream cheese.

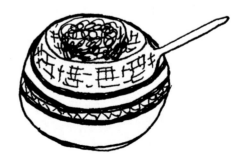

Salmon Spread

15 ounce can salmon
¼ cup fat free mayonnaise
1/8 teaspoon garlic or onion powder
1 tablespoon dried parsley

Remove skin from salmon and discard, mash bones and add to remaining ingredients, mix well. Chill.

Serve with fresh vegetables or low fat crackers or as a filling for sandwiches or as a scoop in a salad or with soup.

4 Servings.

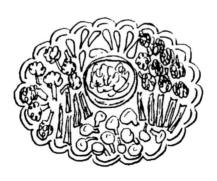

Hungarian Almonds

White from 1 large egg
1 tablespoon paprika
¼ teaspoon ground red pepper (cayenne)
1 teaspoon garlic powder
½ teaspoon salt
2 cups whole almonds with skins on

In a medium bowl beat egg white with a whisk until frothy. Whisk in paprika, red pepper, garlic powder & salt. Add almonds & stir to coat evenly.

Spread on a vegetable sprayed cookie sheet. Bake 25-30 minutes in a 300 degrees oven, stirring occasionally, until lightly toasted. Loosen from pan with spatula. Let cool.

Store airtight.

Makes 2 cups.

6 per serving.

Stuffed Walnuts

3 ounce package fat free cream cheese
72 walnut halves
cinnamon or other seasoning

Put together 2 walnut halves with 1 teaspoon cheese as filling, sprinkled with cinnamon or seasoning of your choice.

These can be frozen. If frozen, thaw desired number of stuffed walnuts in refrigerator about four hours or at room temperature about 1 hour.

Makes 36.   2 per serving.

We cannot direct the wind
but we can adjust our sails

Taco Dip

8 oz. fat-free cream cheese
1 small chopped onion or green onion •
1 large tomato, chopped and seeded
¼ head chopped lettuce
1¼ oz. pkg. taco seasoning mix
4 oz. shredded light cheddar cheese or mozzarella
    or Farmers cheese

Spread cream cheese on large serving plate or platter. Sprinkle lightly with some of the taco seasoning. Layer other ingredients on top of the cheese in order given.

Note: If there seems to be more taco seasoning than you'd like, don't use the whole package. I usually use about ¾ of a package.

6-10 Servings.

No matter where I serve my guests
it seems they like my kitchen best.

Spinach Dip

10 oz. pkg. frozen chopped spinach, thawed and
     pressed or squeezed
3 sliced green onions
8 oz. plain fat free yogurt
1 tablespoon fat free mayonnaise
½ teaspoon onion powder
½ teaspoon salt
1/8 teaspoon pepper

Mix yogurt, mayonnaise and seasonings. Fold in
onions and spinach.

6-8 Servings.

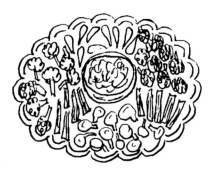

Hot Dried Beef Dip

8 ounces fat free cream cheese
4 ounces fat free sour cream
½ small onion, grated or ¼ teaspoon powdered
      onion
3 ounce package dried beef, chopped
¼ cup chopped pecans
1 teaspoon butter or salad oil

Blend first 4 ingredients, place in shallow oven dish & cover with pecans sauteed in oil or butter.

Bake 20 minutes in 300 degrees oven.

6-8 Servings.

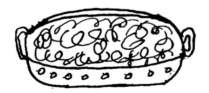

Salsa

2 quarts tomatoes, skinned, seeded &
      coarsely chopped
¾ cup jalapeño peppers, seeded and thinly sliced
1 cup sweet Spanish onions, chopped
1 teaspoon salt
2 tablespoons lemon juice

Bring 1½ quart tomatoes to a boil and slowly simmer until reduced in half (about 2 hours). Stir often to prevent burning. Add the rest of the tomatoes, peppers, onions, salt and lemon juice and
simmer 20 minutes.

10-12 Servings.

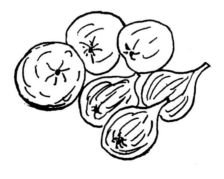

Virgin Mary

3 ounces tomato juice
2 dashes bitter
½ ounce lemon or lime juice
1 dash Worcestershire sauce

Shake together well.

Serve in a tall glass or old fashion glass with ice cubes, garnish with a stalk of celery, lemon or lime slice, wedge or twist.

1 Serving.

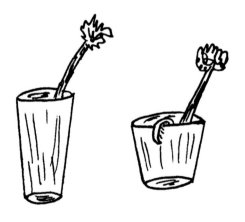

Wine Cooler

1/3 cup white wine
1/3 cup white grape juice (sugar free)
1/3 cup sparkling water

Stir and serve over ice cubes

1 Serving.

Note: Recipe can easily be doubled, tripled etc. Mix in pitcher and add a few thinly sliced lemon or lime and ice cubes.

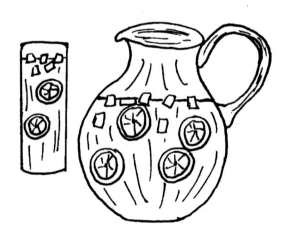

Golden Wassail

4 cups unsweetened pineapple juice
1½ cups apricot nectar (12 ounce can)
4 cups apple juice or apple cider
1 cup orange juice or white grape juice
6 inch stick cinnamon
1 teaspoon whole cloves

Combine all ingredients in a large pan (not aluminum). Heat to boiling point, reduce heat and simmer 15–20 minutes.

Remove from heat, remove cinnamon stick and whole cloves.

Pour hot wassail into mugs.

9 Servings.

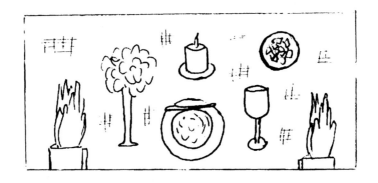

Chapter 2

Breakfast Eggs

French Onion Omelet

1 tablespoon olive oil
2 cups coarsely chopped onions
¼ cup sliced green onions
2 teaspoons Dijon mustard
½ teaspoon dried thyme, crushed
6 eggs or egg substitute
¼ cup water
¼ teaspoon salt
¼ teaspoon white pepper
1 cup shredded Swiss or mozzarella cheese

In a 10 inch ovenproof skillet heat oil over medium heat, add onions, cook for 12-15 minutes or until tender and golden, stirring often. Stir mustard and thyme into skillet.

In bowl beat together eggs, water, salt and pepper. Stir in the cheese. Pour into skillet.

Bake in 375 degrees oven for 10-15 minutes or till set, or on top of stove, covered.

Cut into wedges.

6 Servings.

Pickled Eggs

6 hard cooked eggs, shells removed
1 cup cider vinegar
1 cup liquid drained from canned beets
1 bay leaf
3 whole cloves

Spoon cooked eggs into jar or crock.

Combine cider vinegar and beet liquid, slowly pour down side of jar. Be sure eggs are completely covered by liquid. Add bay leaf and cloves; cover tightly.

Refrigerate 2 or 3 days before serving.

4-6 Servings.

*Blessed is the person who
is too busy to worry in the daytime
and too tired at night.*

Short Cut Soufflé

¼ cup flour
¼ teaspoon salt
1/8 teaspoon white pepper
½ cup mayonnaise
¼ cup milk
1 cup chopped vegetables, flaked fish,
     grated cheese or chopped cooked
     chicken or turkey
4 egg whites

Gently stir flour, salt and pepper into mayonnaise. Do not beat or over mix.

Add milk slowly, stirring until smooth.

Stir in vegetables, cheese, fish or chicken and other seasonings if desired.

Beat egg whites until stiff. Gently fold mayonnaise mixture into egg whites until thoroughly blended.

Pour into greased seven-inch casserole and bake in 325 degrees oven for 40-45 minutes.

4 Servings.

Egg Foo Yung

6 eggs, slightly beaten (or egg substitute)
4 ounce can sliced mushrooms, drained
1 can fancy mixed Chinese vegetables or
      bean sprouts, rinsed and drained
2 teaspoons soy sauce
1/8 teaspoon pepper
3 dashes hot sauce

Mix ingredients.

Using about 1/3 cup scoop put in hot non-stick vegetable sprayed skillet, turn when cooked about half done.

Foo Yung Gravy

1½ cups chicken or vegetable broth
1½ tablespoons cornstarch
1½ teaspoons soy sauce
dash pepper
¼ teaspoon sugar

Blend broth with cornstarch in small saucepan. Stir in soy sauce, pepper & sugar. Cook until mixture thickens & boil 1 minute. 3-4 Servings.

Oven Egg Pancakes

2 large egg whites
2 large eggs or egg substitute
1 cup non fat milk
1/3 cup unbleached all-purpose flour
1 teaspoon sugar
¼ teaspoon salt
¾ cup fat free sour cream

Fruit sauce. Recipe follows.
Preheat oven to 425 degrees.

Beat egg whites in a large bowl until fluffy, continue beating as you add eggs or well shaken egg substitute, then while beating add the milk, flour, sugar and salt. Divide the batter between two glass pie plates, sprayed with vegetable oil. Bake 15 minutes.

When the pancakes are lightly browned, remove from oven and place one pancake on a serving dish. Spread the pancake with sour cream, lightly sprinkle with cinnamon. Top with second pancake. Spoon fruit sauce over top. Cut into wedges.

Fruit Sauce

1¼ cups apple juice
2 tablespoons cornstarch or arrowroot
1 teaspoon vanilla
2 kiwifruits, peeled and cut into large pieces
1 cup frozen blueberries, thawed and drained or
    fresh
1 cup frozen strawberries, thawed and drained or
    fresh

Combine apple juice and cornstarch in a small saucepan, cook over medium heat, stirring. Bring to a boil and cook 1 minute. Add the vanilla, kiwifruits, blueberries and strawberries.
Simmer for 3-5 minutes.

Can prepare ahead of time and reheat.

4 Servings.

It is not good to eat too much honey,
so be sparing with complimentary words.

Easy Egg Omelet

4 ounce container egg substitute
sautéed onions
imitation bacon bits

Sauté onions in a non-stick vegetable sprayed skillet, pour egg substitute, shaken well, over onions, sprinkle with a few imitation bacon bits over the top, cover and cook until done.

3-4 Servings.

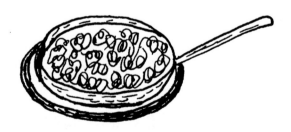

Oven French Toast

3 eggs
½ cup milk
½ teaspoon cinnamon
1/8 teaspoon salt
4 thick slices of bread

Beat eggs, milk, cinnamon and salt in small bowl until frothy.

Place bread in a 9x13 inch baking dish, pour egg mixture over. Refrigerate several hours or overnight, turning once.

Heat on griddle about 5 minutes on each side or heat in preheated 500 degrees oven on a vegetable sprayed baking sheet until golden brown about 5-10 minutes, turning once.

4 Servings.

A memory is a treasure that survives.

Pumpkin Spice Pancakes

1 cup flour
1 tablespoon sugar
1 teaspoon baking powder
½ teaspoon baking soda
½ teaspoon cinnamon
½ teaspoon ginger
½ teaspoon nutmeg
¼ teaspoon salt
¾ cup canned pumpkin
¾ cup milk
½ cup plain fat free yogurt
2 tablespoons vegetable oil
1 large egg

Mix flour, sugar, baking powder, baking soda, cinnamon, ginger, nutmeg and salt.

Whisk pumpkin, milk, yogurt, vegetable oil and egg in a large bowl until blended. Add flour mixture to pumpkin mixture and stir just until mixed, batter will be thick.

Heat griddle or nonstick skillet sprayed with vegetable oil, pour about ¼ cup batter onto griddle. Cook 3-4 minutes until lightly browned and bubbles appear. Turn and cook until lightly browned on bottom. Makes 12 pancakes.

6 Servings.

Pineapple Pancakes

1¼ cups flour
3 teaspoons baking powder
½ teaspoon salt
1 egg, beaten
1 cup milk
2 tablespoons salad oil
½ cup crushed pineapple (in its own juice),
drained

Sift together flour, baking powder and salt. Combine egg, milk and salad oil, add to dry ingredients, stirring just until flour is moistened, (batter will be lumpy). Add the pineapple.

Bake on hot griddle sprayed with vegetable oil, with a scant ¼ cup measure.

Makes 12 pancakes.

4-6 Servings.

Applesauce Oatmeal Pancakes

1 cup quick cooking oatmeal
½ cup flour
1 tablespoon baking powder
¼ teaspoon salt
4 egg whites
3 tablespoons applesauce, unsweetened
2/3 cup milk

In bowl combine the oats, flour, baking powder and salt. Set aside.

In another bowl combine egg whites, slightly beaten with a whisk or fork, add the applesauce and milk. Add to dry ingredients and mix well.

Pour scant ¼ cup batter onto vegetable sprayed heated griddle. Cook until bubbles appear on top, turn and cook until lightly browned.

Spread all fruit jam over the pancakes if desired.

Makes 10 pancakes.

5 Servings.

Breakfast Burritos

6 inch flour tortilla
1 tablespoon all–fruit jam
2 tablespoons low fat raspberry yogurt or choice
Fresh fruit – sliced strawberries, kiwifruit's,
    blueberries, etc.

Spread the tortilla with all fruit jam within ½ inch of edge. Spread with yogurt. Top center third with about 1/4 cup sliced or chopped fruit. Bring edges of tortilla together in the center over lapping slightly. Secure with a tooth pick if needed.

1 Serving.

What we see depends mostly
on what we look for.

Breakfast Bread

2 cups pancake mix
2 tablespoons sugar
¼ cup fat free milk
1 teaspoon vanilla
2 eggs or ½ cup egg substitute
1 cup blueberries

Mix together with a fork. Turn onto floured board and knead lightly. Pat into a 9 inch circle. Cut into 9 or 12 pie shape pieces. Put on vegetable sprayed baking sheet.

Bake in 375 degrees oven 25-30 minutes.

9 Servings.

One who sows courtesy, reaps friendship and one who plants kindness, gathers love.

Quick Oatmeal

¼ cup quick cooking oatmeal
¾ cup water
few raisins

Put oatmeal in a small deep dish, add the water and raisins. Put in the microwave and cook for 2 minutes. Stir. Sprinkle with cinnamon or nutmeg.

Note: Watch that the oatmeal doesn't boil over. That's why you use a deep dish.

1 Serving.

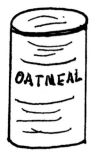 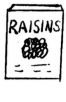

Buttermilk Irish Soda Bread

4 cups all purpose flour
1-1/2 teaspoons baking powder
1 teaspoon baking soda
2 cups buttermilk
2 tablespoons salad oil
1/2 cup raisins

Mix dry ingredients; stir in buttermilk, oil and raisins. Shape into a round loaf and place on a large non-stick pie pan or non-stick cookie sheet or sprayed with cooking oil.

Bake 45-50 minutes in a preheated 350 degree oven.

8-10 Servings.

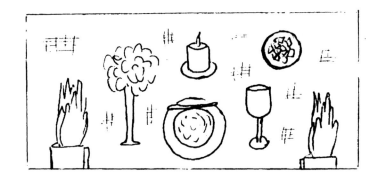

Chapter 3

Salads
Relishes
Sauces

Fresh Strawberry Salad

4 cups red leaf lettuce
1 pint strawberries
2 kiwifruits
¼ cup honey
¼ cup tarragon vinegar
¼ cup salad oil
½ teaspoon dill weed

Wash, dry and tear leaf lettuce. Wash and hull strawberries, quarter. Peel and slice kiwifruits. Toss all gently in bowl.

Combine remaining ingredients. Shake dressing until well mixed.

Just before serving, drizzle dressing over salad ingredients.

4 Servings.

Raspberry Congealed Salad

8 ounce can crushed pineapple
10 ounce package frozen unsweetened
    raspberries, thawed
3 ounce package raspberry gelatin,
    can use sugar free
1 cup unsweetened applesauce
¼ cup coarsely chopped pecans, optional

Drain pineapple, reserving juice. Place pineapple and raspberries in large bowl, set aside.

Add enough water to juice to measure 1 cup, pour into a saucepan, bring to a boil. Remove from heat. Stir in gelatin until dissolved. Pour over fruit mixture. Add the applesauce and pecans. Pour into 1 quart bowl. Chill until set.

Top with a dollop of mayonnaise if desired.

6 Servings.

Everyone smiles in the same language

Red, White & Blue Salad

Oil a 10 inch tube pan or 12 cup Mold

Red Layer
3 ounce package raspberry gelatin,
    can use sugar free
10 ounce frozen strawberries, drained, save liquid

Dissolve raspberry gelatin in ¾ cup boiling water. Add ¾ cup strawberry liquid, adding some water if needed, and the strawberries. Chill until slightly thickened, pour into mold and chill until firm.

White Layer
3 ounce package lemon gelatin, can use sugar free
3 ounce package fat free cream cheese
½ cup fat free sour cream
8 ounces, unsweetened, crushed pineapple,
    drained, save liquid

Dissolved lemon gelatin in ¾ cup boiling water, add ¾ cup pineapple juice, adding water if needed. Chill until slightly thickened. In medium bowl beat cream cheese with sour cream until smooth, stir in lemon gelatin and the drained pineapple, pour over raspberry mixture. Chill until firm.

(Continued on next page)

Blue Layer
3 ounce package black raspberry gelatin,
    can use sugar free
1¼ cups stewed or canned blueberries, drained,
    saving liquid

Dissolve black raspberry gelatin in ¾ cup boiling water, Add 1 cup blueberry juice and blueberries.

Chill until slightly thickened, pour over pineapple mixture. Chill.

To unmold, loosen top with knife. Put mold in warm water and shake slightly until loosen. Unmold.

12 Servings.

Blessed is s/he who scours and scrubs,
for well s/he knows that cleanliness .
is the expression of godliness.

Cottage Cheese Gelatin Salad

3 ounce package lime-flavored gelatin,
      can use sugar free
3 ounce package lemon-flavored gelatin,
      can use sugar free
2 cups boiling water
1 cup evaporated skim milk
juice of one lemon (about 2 tablespoons)
16 ounce can crushed pineapple, drained
16 ounce carton fat free cottage cheese

Combine lime and lemon flavored gelatins, dissolve in boiling water. Cool.

Stir in evaporated milk, lemon juice and drained crushed pineapple. Chill until slightly thickened. Fold in cottage cheese.

Pour into 2 quart bowl or mold or 9x13x2 inch pan.

Chill until firm.

10-12 Servings.

Lettuce Slaw

½ cup fat free sour cream
¼ cup fat free mayonnaise
¼ cup crumbled Roquefort cheese
¼ teaspoon salt
1 tablespoon milk
1 medium head iceberg lettuce
12 cherry tomatoes, stemmed and cut in half
1 cup red beans, drained
2 small white onions, peeled, sliced and
     separated into rings, optional

Combine sour cream, mayonnaise, Roquefort cheese, salt and milk in a small bowl, beat until blended. Chill.

Cut head of lettuce in half, discard core and shred fine. There should be about 8 cups. Place in salad bowl, add tomatoes, beans and onion rings.

Add dressing to lettuce mixture in salad bowl just before serving, toss lightly until evenly mixed.

6 Servings.

Spinach Salad
with Sesame Seed Dressing

2 tablespoons sesame seeds
1/3 cup olive oil
¼ cup lemon juice
2 tablespoons soy sauce
½ teaspoon salt
1/8 teaspoon hot pepper sauce
2 teaspoons brown sugar
¼ pound fresh mushrooms, sliced
8 ounce can sliced water chestnuts
1 pound fresh spinach, torn into large pieces

Heat sesame seeds in saucepan to toast, taking care to avoid burning. Add olive oil, lemon juice, soy sauce, salt, hot pepper sauce and brown sugar. Stir to blend.

Add cleaned and sliced fresh mushrooms and water chestnuts. Marinate overnight. After the mixture sets, it makes its own juice.

Pour over spinach when ready to serve and toss.

Note: Garden lettuce maybe substituted for spinach.

6-8 Servings

Carrot – Raisin Salad

2 cups grated raw carrots
1/3 cup raisins
2 tablespoons fat free mayonnaise
2 tablespoons fat free plain yogurt
1 tablespoon lemon juice
1 teaspoon honey
1/16 teaspoon salt

Combine carrots and raisins

Mix together mayonnaise, yogurt, lemon juice, honey and salt. Pour over salad and mix well. Chill.

4 Servings.

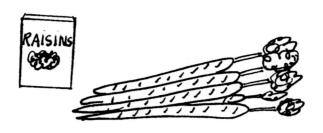

Cranberry Cream Salad

6 ounce package raspberry gelatin,
      can use sugar free
2 cups boiling water
1 can (15 ounces) whole cranberry sauce
2 cups fat free sour cream

Dissolve gelatin in boiling water. Chill until mixture begins to set.

Beat cranberry sauce into gelatin, stir in sour cream. Pour into bowl or mold and chill until set.

6 Servings.

Quick Green Pea Salad

½ cup sour cream
¼ cup, thinly sliced, green onions
¼ teaspoon salt
16 ounce bag frozen green peas,
     thawed and drained
1/16 teaspoon pepper

Mix sour cream, green onions and salt in a serving bowl. Stir in peas and pepper.

Cover and refrigerate until serving time.

4-6 Servings.

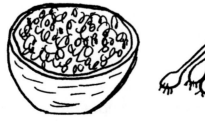
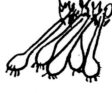

Green Pea Salad

20 ounce package frozen peas
¼ cup fat free mayonnaise
1 tablespoon chopped parsley
1 tablespoon lemon juice
¼ teaspoon salt
1/8 teaspoon pepper

In 3 quart saucepan heat ¾ cup water to boiling, over high heat. Add peas and heat to boiling, reduce heat, cover and simmer 3-5 minutes. Drain peas, rinse under cold water to cool. Drain

Mix mayonnaise, parsley, lemon juice, salt and pepper. Add peas to mayonnaise mixture, toss to coat. Refrigerate.

6 Servings.

*Food kept from going to waste
sometimes goes to waist.*

Easy Green Beans

9 ounce package frozen cut green beans
1 small onion, sliced or chopped
2 tablespoons olive oil and vinegar dressing or
      olive oil and lemon dressing

Steam beans according to the directions on the package. (About 8 minutes) The last two minutes of cooking time left put in the onions and continue cooking. Put beans and onions in dish, stir in dressing while still warm.

Serve warm or as a cold salad.

4 Servings.

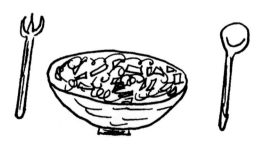

Swedish Green Beans

½ cup fat free sour cream
1/3 cup fat free mayonnaise
16 ounce package frozen French cut green beans,
        cooked or steamed
1 teaspoon dill weed
¼ teaspoon salt
1/8 teaspoon pepper

Blend sour cream, mayonnaise and seasonings.
Pour mixture over cooked vegetables and toss.

Cover and chill for several hours.

4-6 Servings.

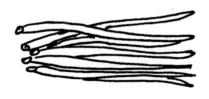

Broccoli Salad

16 ounce package frozen broccoli
½ cup frozen peas
¼ cup stuffed green olives, sliced
¼ cup chopped onions or
       ¼ teaspoon onion powder
¼ cup fat free mayonnaise
¼ cup fat free plain yogurt
¼ teaspoon salt
½ teaspoon dill weed

Steam broccoli for 5 minutes, until bright green and still crisp. Cool. (If broccoli is in large pieces cut into smaller pieces). Steam peas 3-5 minutes. Cool. If using onions steam along with peas the last 2 minutes if desired.

Put broccoli, peas, onions and olives into salad bowl.

Mix mayonnaise, yogurt, salt, dill weed and onion powder, if using, in bowl. Mix dressing into vegetables. Refrigerate 8 hours or overnight.

Before serving lightly sprinkle with more dill weed and about 3 sliced olives for garnish.

6 – 8 Servings.

Fish Salad

16 ounce package frozen cod, thawed
1 cup fat free mayonnaise
½ cup chopped celery, optional
½ cup shredded carrots
½ teaspoon grated onion
2 teaspoon lemon juice
1 package mixed greens or leaf lettuce

Cook fish according to package directions. Cool.
In large bowl, flake cooled fish.

Combine mayonnaise, celery, carrots, grated onion and lemon juice. Mix with flaked fish.
Chill.

Just before serving toss with greens or torn leaf lettuce.

4 Servings.

*It takes both rain and sunshine
to make a rainbow.*

Chicken or Turkey Salad

2 chicken breasts, boneless, skinned and
    cooked or leftover cooked turkey,
    cut into pieces
1 pound frozen mixed vegetables
½ cup fat free mayonnaise
1 tablespoon lemon juice

Steam vegetables 5-7 minutes to desired tenderness.

In large dish, combine chicken or turkey, vegetables and mayonnaise. Add lemon juice and mix well. Chill..

Note: Can add ¼ teaspoon of some herb or seasoned salt, garlic or onion powder.

4-6 Servings.

Life is like a ladder.
Every step we take
is either up or down.

Easy Pasta Salad

16 ounces Bow Tie or other pasta shape
16 ounce bag frozen broccoli, cauliflower
    and carrots or any other combination
1 bunch green onions, cleaned and sliced
1 cup Italian, creamy Italian or
    favorite dressing, low calorie or fat free

Cook pasta according to package directions, drain.

Cook vegetables according to directions, drained (preferably steamed).

Combine drained pasta, vegetables, onions and dressing in a large bowl. Cover and chill until ready to serve.

6-8 Servings.

It's all right to drink like a fish,
if you drink what a fish drinks.

Macaroni Salad

1 pound package small elbow macaroni
1½ cups fat free mayonnaise
1 cup fat free sour cream
3 tablespoons prepared mustard
½ teaspoon salt
1/8 teaspoon pepper
1 medium onion, grated or minced
1 cup finely chopped celery, optional
small jar stuffed green olives, drained and sliced,
    reserving 8 olives, sliced, for garnish

Cook pasta following directions on package, drain. Meanwhile stir together mayonnaise, sour cream, mustard, salt and pepper. Add onion, celery and sliced green olives. Add the pasta, toss to blend well. Cover, refrigerate until ready to serve. (Add additional mayonnaise or sour cream just before serving if salad is too dry). Put salad in salad bowl.

Garnish with the reserved sliced olives.

12 Servings.

Cauliflower and Pea Salad

1 cup fat free mayonnaise
1 package (1 ounce) Ranch style dressing mix
10 ounce package frozen peas
1 head cauliflower, cut into bite size pieces

Mix first 2 ingredients together, set aside.

Steam vegetables 5 minutes. Cool. Mix vegetables with dressing and marinate 8 hours or overnight.

Note: Can also add broccoli, cut into bite size pieces and steamed for 5 minutes, to recipe.

6-8 Servings.

*An open mind
provides the opportunity
for a worthwhile thought to drop in.*

Hearty Bean Salad

2–16 ounce cans red beans, drained
1 small onion, minced
¼ teaspoon salt
¼ cup diced celery
1/8 teaspoon pepper
¼ cup fat free mayonnaise or sour cream

Combine all the ingredients with the mayonnaise or sour cream.

6-8 Servings.

Cranberry Soufflé Salad

1 can cranberry sauce or whole
1 envelope unflavored gelatin
¼ cup fat free mayonnaise

Sprinkle gelatin over cranberries in saucepan. Heat and stir until gelatin is dissolved. Cool.

Fold in mayonnaise. Pour into salad bowl. Chill until firm.

Can pour into 8x5x3 inch loaf pan and slice.

4 Servings.

"Answer not a fool according to his folly,
lest you be like him yourself.
"Answer not a fool according to his folly,
lest he be wise in his own eyes."

Proverbs 26:4-5

Tomato – Onion Salad

1 small red or Spanish onion, cut
        lengthwise in fourths, then sliced
2-3 large tomatoes
¼ teaspoon salt
1 tablespoon olive oil
½ teaspoon basil
1/8 teaspoon pepper, freshly grated

Pour boiling water, to cover, over thinly sliced red onion in small bowl, let stand 5 minutes. Drain well.

Put onion in bowl along with the tomatoes, cut into wedges, add the basil, pepper, salt, and olive oil. Toss lightly.

Note: Peel the tomatoes by putting them in hot water for 1-2 minutes, drain and peel them.

4-6 Servings.

Peas with Fat Free Cream Sauce

1 cup milk
¼ teaspoon salt
1/16 teaspoon white pepper
½ teaspoon onion powder
1 bay leaf
5 ounces freezer peas
2 tablespoons flour
¼ cup water

Heat milk, seasonings and peas. Mix flour and water and stir in until thickened. Remove bay leaf.

Note: Good with a baked potato.

4 Servings.

*S/he who meddles in a quarrel not their own
is like one who
grabs a passing dog by the ears.*

Easy Salad

½ head lettuce or other greens, cleaned
tomato or cherry tomatoes or
      small yellow pear tomatoes
salad dressing
garlic

Cut garlic clove in half, rub inside of salad bowl with cut side garlic.

Break up lettuce and tear into bite size pieces, put in bowl, add tomato, cut into wedges or cherry tomatoes or yellow pear tomatoes or both, cut in half.

Refrigerate if making early in the day.

Just before serving toss with your favorite salad dressing or with Italian salad dressing using 3 parts olive oil and 1 part wine vinegar or lemon juice, salt and pepper to taste.

4 Servings.

S/he who laughs ... lasts.

Kraut Relish

15 ounce can sauerkraut, drained
¼ cup canned pimento, chopped
½ cup fat free mayonnaise
1 tablespoon prepared horseradish, optional
1/8 teaspoon nutmeg
1/16 teaspoon cayenne pepper

Put drained sauerkraut and chopped pimento into a bowl.

Combine mayonnaise, horseradish, nutmeg and cayenne pepper. Stir into kraut mixture and mix well. Chill.

4-6 Servings.

Refusing to ask for help when you need it
is refusing someone the chance to be helpful.

Creamed Green Peas

16 ounce package frozen green peas
¼ cup fat free mayonnaise
1 teaspoon lemon juice
¼ teaspoon salt
1/8 teaspoon pepper

Steam peas about 5 minutes. Cool.

Mix mayonnaise, lemon juice, salt and pepper.
Stir in cooled peas.

4-6 Servings.

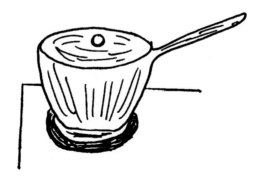

Kidney Bean Salad

16 ounce can kidney or
     red beans, rinsed and drained
¼ cup fat free mayonnaise
¼ teaspoon onion powder or
     ½ teaspoon minced dry onions
1/16 teaspoon pepper

Mix mayonnaise, onion powder and pepper. Mix with beans.

4-6 Servings.

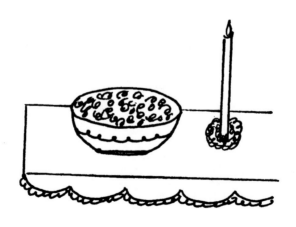

Creamed Beets

15 ounce can diced beets, drained
¼ cup fat free mayonnaise
1 teaspoon Dijon mustard
1 teaspoon horseradish
1 tablespoon water

Mix mayonnaise, mustard, horseradish and water.
Mix with beets.

4 Servings.

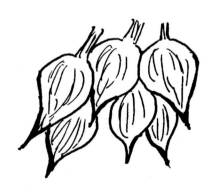

Creamed Green Beans

15 ounce can cut or French cut green beans,
     drained or 2 cups frozen green beans;
     steamed
¼ cup fat free mayonnaise
1 teaspoon grated onion
1 tablespoon milk

Mix mayonnaise, onion juice and milk. Add to green beans.

4 Servings.

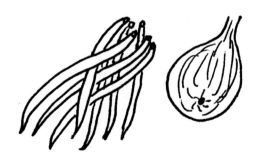

Creamed Red Cabbage

16 ounce jar sweet and sour red cabbage, drained
¼-½ cup fat free sour cream (or to taste)

Add sour cream to the drained cabbage, heat or serve cold.

4 Servings.

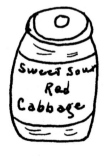 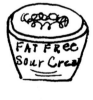

Corn Relish

¼ cup sweet pickle relish
1 tablespoon cornstarch
1 teaspoon turmeric
2 tablespoons wine vinegar
¼ cup water
11 ounce can vacuum packed whole kernel corn,
      drained or 1½ cups frozen corn, steamed

Combine ingredients in a saucepan. Cook and stir over medium heat until mixture thickens. Chill.

4 Servings.

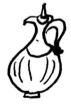
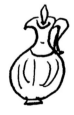

Mock Hollandaise

½ cup fat free mayonnaise
½ teaspoon Dijon mustard
1 teaspoon lemon juice
1/16 teaspoon red pepper

Mix ingredients.

Drizzle sauce over steamed broccoli, cauliflower or asparagus.

4-6 Servings.

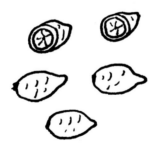

Fat Free Cream Sauce

1 cup milk
¼ teaspoon salt
½ teaspoon onion powder
¼ teaspoon dried thyme
½ bay leaf
2 tablespoons flour
¼ cup water

Heat milk and seasonings. Mix flour and water, stir in until thickened. Remove bay leaf.

4-6 Servings.

Yogurt – Dill Sauce

½ cup fat free plain yogurt
¼ cup fat free mayonnaise
1 teaspoon dried dill weed
½ teaspoon Dijon mustard

Combine all ingredients and mix well.

Use as sauce for vegetables, salads or as a dip.

Yield ¾ cup.

Note: Heat if desired, but do not allow to boil.

2 Tablespoons per serving.

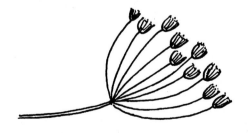

Oil and Lemon Dressing

3 tablespoons olive or canola oil
2 tablespoons lemon juice
½ teaspoon crushed dried basil
¼ teaspoon fresh ground pepper
1 clove garlic, peeled
½ teaspoon salt, optional

Combined all ingredients in a covered glass jar, shake well and set aside.

At serving time remove the clove of garlic.

Dressing can be made a day or so ahead. Refrigerate.

Combine with mixed greens and vegetables or steamed vegetables.

2 Tablespoons per serving.

*Well-timed silence
has more eloquence than speech.*

Fruit Sauce

1¼ cups apple juice
2 tablespoons cornstarch or arrowroot
1 teaspoon vanilla
2 kiwifruits, peeled and cut into large pieces
1 cup frozen blueberries, thawed and drained or
     fresh
1 cup frozen strawberries, thawed and drained or
     fresh

Combine apple juice and cornstarch in a small saucepan, cook over medium heat, stirring. Bring to a boil and cook 1 minute. Add the vanilla, kiwifruit's, blueberries and strawberries.
Simmer for 3-5 minutes.

Can prepare ahead of time and reheat.

4 Servings.

It is not good to eat too much honey,
so be sparing with complimentary words.

Garlic Puree

2 whole flowers garlic, peeled
3 tablespoons olive oil

In food processor add garlic, run and add olive oil, through the tube, until a fine paste.

Use ½ teaspoon to equal 1 clove garlic.

Refrigerate.

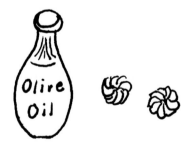

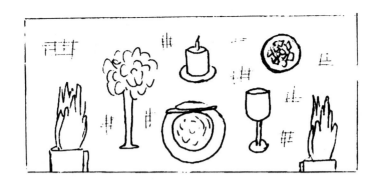

Chapter 4

Soups

Quick Cream of Broccoli Soup

½ cup onions, coarsely chopped
2½ cups broth, vegetable or chicken or turkey
16 ounce package frozen broccoli
1 cup fat free milk

Bring to a boil in saucepan onion, broth and broccoli. Lower heat and simmer 10 minutes covered.
Puree in blender with some of the milk if needed.
Put back in pan, add milk, and simmer a few minutes until heated through.

When serving, sprinkle with a little nutmeg or a
dollop of fat free sour cream or yogurt.

4-6 Servings.

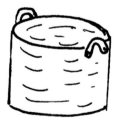
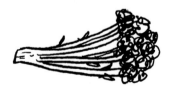

Zucchini Soup

2 – 3 medium zucchinis, about 12 ounces,
      coarsely chopped
½ cup chopped onion
1 clove garlic, crushed or ½ teaspoon puree
½ teaspoon curry powder
¾ cup vegetable broth
1 cup fat free milk

Put onion, garlic, curry powder, zucchini and broth in saucepan. Bring to boil, simmer, covered for 15 minutes.

Puree in blender with some of the milk if needed, return to saucepan, add milk and heat through.

When serving swirl 1 teaspoon of yogurt in soup.

4 Servings.

Head cold: rheum at the top.

Curried Squash Soup

2 packages (12 ounces each) frozen cooked
      winter squash
2 cups broth, vegetable
2/3 cup fat free milk
½ teaspoon onion powder
½ teaspoon curry powder
1/8 teaspoon salt

Heat frozen squash and broth in a covered 3 quart saucepan over medium heat, about 5 minutes, stirring once or twice until squash is thawed.

Stir in milk, onion powder, curry powder and salt. Heat through for flavors to develop.

4-6 Servings.

Some minds are like concrete:
all mixed up and permanently set.

Squash Soup

¾ cup celery, sliced thin
½ cup chopped onion
¾ cup sliced carrot, can use frozen
3 cups broth, vegetable, chicken or turkey
12 ounce package frozen cooked winter squash,
        thawed
1/8 teaspoon ground cloves
¼ teaspoon salt
½ teaspoon ginger

Simmer vegetables in one cup broth in saucepan, covered, about 15-20 minutes. Add thawed squash, seasonings and rest of broth. Heat thoroughly.

4 Servings.

Thank God for dirty dishes,
they have a tale to tell.
While others suffer hunger,
we're eating pretty well.
With home and health and happiness
I shouldn't want to fuss;
for by this stack of evidence,
God's very good to us.

Cream of Asparagus Soup

2 – 8 ounce packages frozen asparagus or
    1½ pounds fresh asparagus
1 small onion, coarsely chopped
2 cups vegetable broth or choice of broth
1½ cups fat free milk
1/8 teaspoon nutmeg
1/16 teaspoon white pepper, optional

Thaw asparagus. Remove tips, put aside. In saucepan combine broth, asparagus and onion. Bring to a boil over medium heat, reduce heat, cover and simmer about 12 – 15 minutes.

Meanwhile cook tips in small amount of water in microwave about 1 – 2 minutes.

Put cooked asparagus mixture in blender and blend until smooth. Put back in saucepan along with milk, nutmeg and pepper. Heat until hot.

Serve in bowls garnished with asparagus tips.

4-6 Servings.

Forty is the old age of youth;
Fifty is the youth of old age.

Cream of Parsley and Basil Soup

1 bunch parsley, stems removed (about 4 cups)
½ cup basil, stems removed
2½ cups stock or broth
1 large potato, peeled and cut into chunks
12 ounces evaporated skim milk
1/16 teaspoon pepper
1/16 teaspoon nutmeg
2 tablespoons flour mixed with ¼ cup water

Put stock, potato, parsley and basil into saucepan.
Bring to a boil, cover and simmer for 20 minutes.
Allow mixture to cool slightly. Puree in blender
or food processor until smooth.

Return to saucepan; add milk, pepper and nutmeg.
Heat thoroughly. Stir in flour and water mixture,
stir until thickened.

Garnish each bowl with basil leaf.

6 Servings.

When both intuition and logic agree,
we're quite likely right.

Cream of Parsley Soup

1 bunch parsley, stems removed, about 4 cups
1 small onion, coarsely chopped
2½ cups vegetable broth or choice
12 ounces evaporated skim milk
1/16 teaspoon pepper
1/16 teaspoon nutmeg
3 tablespoons flour mixed with ¼ cup water

Put broth, onion and parsley in saucepan. Bring to boil. Cover and simmer 20 minutes. Allow mixture to cool slightly. Puree in blender until smooth. Return mixture to saucepan, add milk, pepper and nutmeg. Heat, stir in flour and water mixture, stir until thickened.

Garnish each bowl with a parsley sprig or sprinkle lightly with nutmeg.

4-6 Servings.

*The greatest remedy for anger
is delay.*

Spinach – Celery Soup

2 ribs celery
1 small yellow onion, coarsely chopped
3 cups broth
1 small potato, diced or
     1½ cups frozen hash browns
10 ounce package frozen spinach, thawed
½ teaspoon nutmeg
½ teaspoon salt (optional)
1/16 teaspoon pepper
1½ cups milk

Put broth, celery, onion and potato in saucepan bring to a boil and simmer, covered, for 20-30 minutes. Add spinach, nutmeg, salt and pepper. Simmer 1-2 minutes more.

Remove from heat; puree half of mixture until smooth in blender or food processor. Pour into a bowl, puree rest of mixture and pour all back into saucepan, add milk and reheat.

4-6 Servings.

Spinach Soup

10 ounce package frozen chopped spinach,
       thawed
3 tablespoons flour
½ small onion, coarsely chopped
1½ cups vegetable broth or choice
1/8 teaspoon nutmeg
¼ teaspoon salt, optional
1/16 teaspoon freshly ground pepper
1 cup milk

Put spinach, onion and broth in sauce pan, cook 10 minutes.

Put spinach mixture and some of the milk, if needed, in blender after cooling somewhat and puree. Put back in saucepan, add seasonings and flour mixed with some of the milk and remaining milk. Heat until smooth and thickened.

4 Servings.

Salesmanship starts when the customer says "no."

Tomato - Cabbage Soup

46 ounces tomato juice
2 teaspoons vegetable broth base dissolved in
½ cup hot water
½ teaspoon oregano
½ teaspoon basil
1 package cabbage coleslaw

Combine all ingredients, except cabbage, bring to a boil. Add shredded cabbage and heat thoroughly, about 5 minutes.

Note: Can use a small head cabbage if you desire, but not in the food processor, it gets too fine. Also can cut the packaged coleslaw a little finer, if you like.

6-8 Servings.

The first great gift we can bestow on others is a good example.

Cabbage Soup With Roquefort

2 ½ pound head cabbage, cored, quartered
     and coarsely chopped (discard the core)
1 large onion, coarsely chopped
1 teaspoon salt
¼ cup oil
cooked, smoked, ham hock
3 cups broth
3 cups water
¼ cup milk
2 tablespoons Roquefort cheese

In large saucepan, cook the cabbage, onion, salt and oil over moderate heat for 30 minutes or until the vegetables are soft. Add the cooked ham hock, broth and water. Bring to a boil, lower heat and simmer 25 minutes.

Shred the ham hock and add to the soup.

In small bowl whisk the milk into the Roquefort cheese until well softened and stir the mixture into the soup. Season with pepper to taste if needed.

6-8 Servings.

Cauliflower Soup

Small head of cauliflower, cut off stem and outer leaves and discard, break cauliflower into pieces. Or can use 16 ounce package of frozen cauliflower

½ teaspoon salt, optional
1½ teaspoons lemon juice
1 small onion, coarsely chopped
2 cups water
2 cups vegetable broth
1/16 teaspoon white pepper
1/8 teaspoon nutmeg

Combine cauliflower, salt, lemon juice, onion, water and vegetable broth in saucepan. Simmer 20-25 minutes.

Puree in blender until smooth. Return to saucepan add pepper and nutmeg and reheat.

In serving bowl sprinkle lightly with nutmeg.

Note: Can add ¾ cup milk to the soup if desired. Add after you puree in the blender.

6 Servings.

Carrot Bisque

3 cups broth, vegetable, turkey or chicken
16 ounce package freezer carrots or fresh cut in
    rounds
1 medium onion, coarsely chopped
¼ cup smooth peanut butter
1/8 teaspoon cayenne pepper, optional

In saucepan combine broth, carrots and onions. Bring to boil over high heat, reduce heat to low and simmer, covered, until vegetables are tender, about 30 minutes. Put contents into blender and puree. In small bowl mix ½ cup puree with peanut butter and cayenne pepper until well combined.

In saucepan blend peanut butter mixture and remaining puree. Cover and simmer until heated through, about 5 minutes.

Garnish with croutons if desired.

Serve hot or cold.

4 Servings.

One of the rarest things we do
is the best we can.

Carrot Soup

1 medium onion, chopped
2 cups potatoes, diced or freezer hash browns
16 ounce package freezer carrots or fresh
5 cups broth
1 teaspoon summer savory
1 teaspoon basil
1/8 teaspoon pepper
1 cup milk

In saucepan put onion, carrots, potatoes, broth and seasonings. Bring to boil over high heat, reduce heat to low and simmer, covered, 20-30 minutes until vegetables are tender. Cool slightly. Puree in blender until very smooth. Return to saucepan and reheat. Stir in milk and heat but do not boil.

Ladle into soup bowls and lightly sprinkle with nutmeg.

4-6 Servings.

Sometimes the best thing to get off our chest is our chin.

Cream of Vegetable Soup
(Quickie)

4 cups frozen hash brown potatoes, thawed
1½ cups frozen diced carrots and peas, thawed
1 cup frozen cut green beans, thawed
½ cup chopped onion
½ teaspoon dried basil
½ teaspoon dried thyme
1 bay leaf
5 cups broth
2/3 cup non fat dry milk
½ cup instant potato flakes

Place all ingredients in soup kettle, except dry milk and instant potato flakes, bring to a boil and simmer, covered, 15-20 minutes or until vegetables are tender. Remove bay leaf, add dry milk and instant potato flakes. Stir until flakes are dissolved.

Note: If you just want a plain vegetable soup eliminate the powdered milk and instant potatoes.

6 Servings.

Chunky Vegetable Soup

1 medium onion, chopped
1 package cabbage–carrot coleslaw
4 cups broth
3 cups water
1 teaspoon dried basil
½ teaspoon dried oregano
2 medium size zucchinis, sliced, about 12 ounces
1 cup macaroni

In soup kettle, put broth, cabbage-carrot mixture, onions, water, basil and oregano. Bring to boil over high heat, reduce heat, cover and simmer 20-30 minutes. Increase heat, add zucchini and pasta, bring to boil, cover, reduce heat and simmer 10-12 minutes longer or until pasta is tender.

6 Servings.

Humor is the hole that lets the sawdust out of a stuffed shirt.

Cabbage - Bean Soup

4 cups vegetable broth
1 cup water
small head cabbage, coarsely chopped
1½ cups sliced carrots
1 cup sliced onion
½ teaspoon ground cloves
2 – 15 ounce cans navy beans
2 teaspoons dill weed

Bring broth, water, cabbage, carrots and onions to a boil in large pot. Reduce heat, cover, and simmer 12 minutes until vegetables are firm tender. Add beans, dill weed and cloves, simmer, uncovered, 5 minutes.

Garnish with a dollop of sour cream and dill weed.

4-6 Servings.

Opportunities are seldom labeled.

Kale – Potato Soup

4 cups broth
2 medium onions, coarsely chopped
5 or 6 ounces kale
¾ cup potato flakes
1/8 teaspoon pepper
1/8 teaspoon nutmeg
1/3 cup dry milk

Bring broth, onions and kale to a boil, simmer, covered, about 10 minutes.

Puree half the mixture at a time in a blender and return to saucepan. Stir in dry milk, potato flakes, pepper and nutmeg.

Note: Can use spinach in place of kale.

6 Servings.

*The human spirit is stronger than anything
that can happen to it.*

Spinach – Rice Soup

2 medium onions, peeled and coarsely chopped
6½ cups broth
½ cup rice
2 – 10 ounce packages frozen, chopped spinach,
    thawed
½ teaspoon salt
¼ teaspoon nutmeg
1/8 teaspoon pepper

Bring broth and onions to a boil, add rice and boil, uncovered, 10 minutes. Add remaining ingredients and simmer 12-15 minutes longer until rice is done.

6-8 Servings.

*The most effective way to cope with change
is to help create it.*

Pureed Vegetable Soup

16 ounce package freezer broccoli
    and cauliflower mix
4 cups broth
1 medium onion, chopped
1 bay leaf
1/2 teaspoon dried basil
1/2 teaspoon dried thyme

In saucepan, bring broccoli and cauliflower, broth, onion and bay leaf to a boil, lower heat and simmer, covered, for 20 minutes until vegetables are tender. Stir in herbs. Let cool for a few minutes. Remove bay leaf.

Puree in blender or food processor until smooth. Put back in saucepan and heat through.

Garnish with ½ inch sliced green onion.

4 Servings.

*The best effect of the energy crisis
is the renewed use of elbow grease.*

White Bean and Carrot Soup

1 tablespoon olive oil
1 medium onion, chopped
2 cloves garlic, finely chopped or
       ¼ teaspoon powdered
2 – 19 ounce cans navy beans, drained and rinsed
¾ teaspoon dried thyme, crumbled
10 ounce package frozen sliced carrots, thawed
14½ ounce can reduced–sodium broth

Heat oil in medium size saucepan. Add onion and garlic, cook 5 minutes. Add half the beans, thyme, carrots and broth, cook 5 minutes or until carrots are tender.

Meanwhile puree remaining beans in blender or food processor. Stir into soup, heat through.

4 Servings.

We often discover what will do
by finding out what will not do.

Pumpkin and Bean Soup

2 tablespoons olive oil
1 small onion, chopped
1 garlic clove, minced
29 ounce can pumpkin
2 cups broth
½ cup water
½ teaspoon oregano
¼ teaspoon curry powder
1/8 teaspoon pepper
1 bay leaf
16 ounce can tomatoes, with liquid
3 ounces Canadian bacon, sliced ¼ inch thick and
        cut into quarters
17 ounce can cannellini beans
1 tablespoon dried parsley
½ teaspoon salt

In large soup pot, heat olive oil over low heat, add onion and garlic, cook gently until softened, about 5 minutes. Add pumpkin, broth, water, oregano, curry powder, pepper and bay leaf. Bring to boil, reduce heat and simmer, covered, for 5 minutes. Add the tomatoes, bacon, beans, parsley and salt. Heat through.

Remove bay leaf and serve.

6 Servings

Pasta and Cauliflower Soup

¾ cup sliced frozen carrots or fresh
¼ cup chopped onions
2 cups cauliflower florets
¾ cup small pasta shells
1 tablespoon chopped fresh basil or
        1 teaspoon dried
¼ teaspoon salt
1/16 teaspoon pepper

Bring 5 cups water to a boil, add carrots, onions and cauliflower, cover and cook 5 minutes. Stir in shells, basil and salt. Bring to a boil, lower heat and simmer 10–12 minutes or until shells are tender. Season with pepper.

4 Servings.

Most people put on weight in certain places,
like doughnut shops.

Chunky Cream of Potato Soup

2 – 15 ounce cans whole potatoes, drained
2½ cups chicken or turkey broth
1 cup chopped onions
2/3 cup chopped celery, optional
½ teaspoon dried dill weed
2 cups milk

Combine half potatoes with broth, onions, celery and dill weed in large saucepan. Cover and bring to a boil, reduce heat and simmer, covered, until celery is tender, about 15 minutes. Remove from heat and cool slightly. Ladle half of soup into blender or food processor and puree until smooth. Put mixture in bowl and repeat with remaining soup mixture. Return pureed soup to saucepan.

Cut remaining potatoes into bite-size pieces. Add to soup. Stir in milk and heat through, about 5 minutes. Serve hot.

Can be prepared a day ahead. Cover and refrigerate. Warm over medium heat before serving.

6 Servings.

Potato Soup

½ cup chopped or sliced carrots, can use frozen
½ cup chopped celery
½ cup chopped onion
3½ cups broth, vegetable, turkey or chicken
1 cup fat-free milk
1½ cups instant potato flakes or buds

In large saucepan bring carrots, celery, onion, and broth to a boil, cover. Reduce heat and simmer until vegetables are crispy tender, about 15 minutes.

Stir in milk and potato flakes. Heat through.

Garnish with chives or sprinkle lightly with dill weed.

Note: Can substitute 1 cup freezer sweet peas for the celery or just add the peas, thawed, to the soup when you add the milk.

4 Servings.

Life is like an onion: we peel it off layer by layer, and sometimes we weep.

Easy Potato Soup

1 tablespoon olive oil or choice
½ cup chopped onions
4 cups milk
15 ounce can sliced potatoes, drained
1 cup instant potato flakes
½ teaspoon salt
1/16 teaspoon white pepper

Put oil in saucepan, add chopped onion and cook until soft. Add 4 cups milk and the potatoes cook over medium heat, until milk is hot, but not boiling. Turn off heat and stir in 1 cup of potato flakes or to desired consistency. Season with salt and pepper.

4 Servings

Too many people itch
for what they want,
without being willing
to scratch for it.

French Onion Soup

4 large onions
2 tablespoons olive oil
½ teaspoon salt
1/8 teaspoon pepper
¼ cup dry white wine or dry vermouth
1 quart broth
French bread or purchased croutons
Parmesan cheese, grated

Cut peeled onions in half lengthwise then slice crosswise in thin slices.

Put oil in saucepan and heat. Add onions, salt and pepper. Turn heat to medium and stir occasionally. When onions start to brown, add the wine; cook until onions are caramel color. Add broth. Simmer and adjust seasonings.

When serving soup, make croutons from French bread or purchased croutons and put over soup. Sprinkle with the Parmesan cheese if desired, can put in heatproof bowl and put in oven for cheese to melt.

4-6 Servings.

Cream of Onion Soup

3 cups sliced onions
½ teaspoon salt
½ cup chopped celery
1 cup broth
1/8 teaspoon pepper
1/8 teaspoon nutmeg
1 cup nonfat dry milk
2 tablespoons flour

In large saucepan, bring 4 cups water, salt, onions and celery to a boil. Cook until onions are tender, about 25 minutes. Puree in blender until smooth. Pour back into saucepan and add broth, pepper, nutmeg, nonfat dry milk and flour mixed in ¼ cup water. Cook over low heat until slightly thickened, stirring constantly and heat thoroughly. Do not allow to boil.

Sprinkle lightly with mace or nutmeg

6 Servings.

Diplomacy: the art of letting someone else have your way.

Sweet Pea Soup

1 tablespoon oil
1 medium yellow onion, chopped
¼ teaspoon dill weed
½ teaspoon salt
1/16 teaspoon freshly ground black pepper
16 ounces frozen sweet peas
2 cups milk

In large saucepan, heat oil over medium heat. Add onions and sauté without browning them for about 5 minutes. Add remaining ingredients, bring to a boil and remove from heat. Puree in blender half of mixture until smooth, put in bowl and puree the rest of ingredients. Return to saucepan and reheat over medium-low heat.

Garnish with a dollop of sour cream lightly sprinkled with dill weed.

4-6 Servings.

A book shut is a block of wood.

Tomato Soup

3 cups vegetable broth or choice
6 ounces tomato paste
1/3 cup milk
1 bay leaf
1 teaspoon honey, optional

Bring broth to a boil; add tomato paste and stir. Add milk, honey and bay leaf. Bring to a boil. Remove bay leaf and serve.

Serve with croutons or small dollop of sour cream.

3-4 Servings.

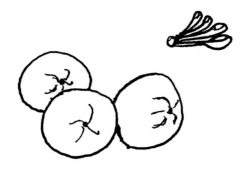

Pumpkin Bisque

29 ounce can pumpkin
2 cups vegetable broth or choice
¼ teaspoon nutmeg
¼ teaspoon cinnamon
½ teaspoon ginger
12 ounce can evaporated skim milk

Place all ingredients, except the evaporated skim milk, in a large saucepan. Bring to a boil and simmer 8 – 10 minutes. Stir in evaporated milk and heat through.

Garnish: Sprinkle lightly with cinnamon or a dollop of sour cream or yogurt and sprinkle with cinnamon lightly.

4 Servings.

Nothing so needs reforming
as other people's habits.

Celery Soup

2 cups celery
½ cup chopped onion
½ cup peeled and diced potato
2 tablespoons minced fresh parsley leaves
1 garlic clove, crushed
2 tablespoons oil
2 cups broth – turkey, vegetable or chicken
1/16 teaspoon pepper
yogurt, plain

In large saucepan simmer celery, onion, potato, parsley, garlic clove in oil, covered, over moderate heat for 20 minutes or until vegetables are soft.

Add broth and bring to a boil. Add pepper.

Puree half the mixture in a blender until smooth. Put in a bowl and puree the other half. Transfer the mixture to saucepan. Heat soup until it is hot.

Ladle into bowls and garnish with a dollop of yogurt.

4-6 Servings.

Navy Bean Soup

16 ounce package dried navy beans
7 cups water
1 bay leaf
16 ounces ham, cubed
1 cup chopped onions
2 stalks celery, cut up
½ cup chopped carrots

Rinse beans. Heat beans and water to boiling. Remove from heat, cover, let stand 1 hour. Add remaining ingredients, heat to boiling, reduce heat and simmer 1½ hours or until beans are soft. Skim off foam occasionally, Season with salt and pepper if needed. Remove bay leaf and mash part of the soup ingredients if desired.

6-8 Servings.

*Only one who can see the invisible
can do the impossible.*

Peanut Soup

2 tablespoons vegetable oil
¾ cup creamy peanut butter
3 cups broth
salt and pepper to taste

Heat oil in saucepan, blend in peanut butter.

Add broth slowly, stirring constantly until mixture is smooth. Bring to a boil, season and lower heat, simmer 10 minutes.

Garnish with freshly ground pepper or croutons.

4-5 Servings

The bigger a person's head gets,
the easier it is to fill their shoes.

131

Egg Drop Soup

1 egg, well beaten
4 cups broth, boiling
chopped parsley

Slowly pour 1 well beaten egg into 4 cups boiling broth, stirring constantly.

Garnish with chopped parsley.

6 Servings

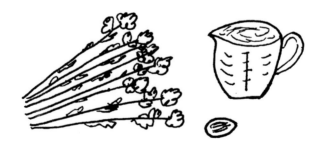

Wild Rice Soup

2 tablespoons oil
¼ cup minced onion
¼ cup flour
3 cups broth
2 cups cooked wild rice
¼ teaspoon salt
1 cup evaporated skim milk
2 tablespoons dry sherry, optional

Heat oil in 3 quart saucepan. Sauté onion until tender. Blend in flour, gradually add broth. Cook stirring constantly until thick.

Stir in wild rice and salt. Simmer 5 minutes, blend in evaporated milk and sherry if desired. Heat until hot, but do not boil.

6 Servings

*A good memory is one that is trained
to forget the trivial.*

Hearty Lentil Soup

3 carrots, sliced – can use frozen carrots
1 medium onion, chopped
1 clove garlic, minced
1 bay leaf
1 cup dry lentils
16 ounce can stewed tomatoes
½ teaspoon salt
1 teaspoon thyme leaves
1/8 teaspoon pepper
½ pound kielbasa, optional
1 tablespoon lemon juice

In 3 quart saucepan, cook carrots, onions, garlic, bay leaf, lentils, tomatoes, salt, thyme, pepper and 5 cups water, covered for 40-50 minute until lentils are tender. Stir a couple times. Slice kielbasa, stir into soup, cook covered for 5 minutes. Stir in lemon juice. Let stand 5 minute. Remove bay leaf.

Note: I usually sauté kielbasa after slicing, in a non-stick skillet to get most of the fat out. It also gives them a better flavor.

6 Servings.

Turkey Chowder

¼ cup chopped onions
1 cup diced celery
2 cups cubed potatoes
1 cup diced cooked turkey
2 cups turkey broth
2 tablespoons chopped parsley
2 tablespoons flour
1 cup milk
1/2 teaspoon salt
1/8 teaspoon pepper

In a 3 quart saucepan cook onions, celery, potatoes, turkey and broth until vegetables are tender. Add parsley.

Blend flour with milk and stir into cooking mixture. Cook about 15 minutes longer, stirring occasionally. Season to taste.

6 Servings.

*It is easier to do a job right
than to explain why we didn't.*

Chicken and Corn Soup

2 boneless, skinless chicken breast or
      turkey, cooked and cubed
¼ cup ham, cubed
16 ounce can cream style corn
6 cups chicken broth
2 tablespoons cornstarch
2 tablespoons water
soy sauce
white pepper

Put chicken, ham, corn and broth in a sauce pan, bring to a boil, simmer about 5 minutes.

Mix cornstarch and water, add to soup mixture and simmer about 5 more minutes.

Season with a little soy sauce and white pepper, according to your taste.

6 Servings.

Inhibitions are tied up in nots.

Quick Noodle Vegetable Soup

3 cups broth
2 cups water
6 ounces medium shells or bows or
     choice of noodles
8 ounces frozen Oriental-style vegetables, thawed
1 tablespoon soy sauce

Bring broth and water to a boil, add the noodles and cook until almost tender, about 7 minutes. Stir in the thawed vegetables. Cook about 5-7 minutes or until vegetables are crisp tender. Season with the soy sauce.

4 Servings.

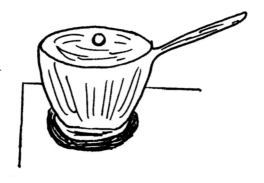

India Lentil Soup

¾ cup dried lentils
2 cups broth
1 medium onion, chopped
1/8 teaspoon chili powder
1½ teaspoons curry powder
1/8 teaspoon ginger powder
1 teaspoon lime or lemon juice

Soak lentils in water, to cover, for 1 hour. Drain
Bring broth and 1 quart of water to boil. Add lentils and cook over low heat 15 minutes. Add the
chopped onions, chili powder, curry and ginger
and cook 15 minutes. Add the lime or lemon juice
and cook about 5 minutes more. Taste for seasoning.

Garnish with chopped parsley if desired.

4 Servings.

Lost time is never found.

Garlic Soup

2 tablespoons olive oil
1 pound onions, coarsely chopped
2 heads garlic (about 28 garlic cloves)
     remove skins and slice
3 cups broth or stock
3 ounces French bread or
     4 slices white bread, torn into pieces
5 parsley sprigs or 1 tablespoon dried
1 teaspoon thyme
½ bay leaf or 1 small
½ teaspoon salt
¼ teaspoon pepper
1 cup fat free milk

Heat olive oil in large saucepan, add onions and garlic, cook until onions are tender and golden brown, stirring frequently, about 30 minutes.

Add to saucepan broth, bread and seasonings. Bring to boil, reduce heat and simmer 15 minutes. Remove bay leaf. Puree mixture in batches in blender. Transfer mixture to large saucepan. Mix in milk and heat.

4-6 Servings.

Dill Pickle Soup

2 tablespoons oil
1 small onion, chopped
4 cups water
1½ cups marinade from pickles
3 large dill pickles, cut into chunks
½ cup white wine
2 teaspoons dried dill weed
¾ teaspoon poultry seasoning
½ teaspoon salt
1/8 teaspoon white pepper
1/3 cup flour

Heat oil in large soup kettle over medium heat, add onion and sauté until soft, add water, pickle juice and dill pickles, simmer about 5 minutes. Cool slightly, puree half mixture in blender, put in a dish, and puree remaining mixture. Put all in soup kettle along with wine, dill weed, poultry seasoning, salt and pepper. Bring to a boil.

Mix the 1/3 cup flour with 1 cup water and add to the soup mixture, stirring until thickened.

Garnish each serving with diced pickles or and dill weed.

6-8 Servings.

Note: Stir in some powdered milk if a lighter color is desired.

Sweet Potato Soup

1 medium onion, sliced
¼ cup water
2 cloves garlic, sliced
2 stalks celery, sliced
¾ teaspoon dried thyme
3 cups broth
2½ cups sliced, peeled sweet potatoes,
    (about 2 large)
2½ cups sliced, peeled russet potatoes,
    (about 2 large)
1 cup fat free milk
2 tablespoons sliced green onions

Combine onion, water and garlic in soup kettle. Cover, cook over low heat until water evaporates and onion is tender, stirring frequently about 8 minutes. Add celery, thyme, broth and all potatoes, bring to a boil. Reduce heat to medium low, cover and simmer until potatoes are tender, about 25 minutes.

Puree mixture in blender or processor in batches. Return puree to pot. Add milk and simmer over low heat until heated through.
Season to taste with salt and pepper if needed.
Garnish each bowl with sliced green onions.

6 Servings.

Note: Can be made 1 day ahead. Cover and refrigerate. Reheat over medium heat.

Corn Chowder

16 ounce package whole kernel corn
4 ounce can green chilies, drained
3 cups broth
1 cup non fat dry milk powder
¼ teaspoon salt
¼ teaspoon pepper

Combine 3 cups of the corn, green chilies and 1 cup broth in blender. Puree until smooth. Pour corn puree mixture into saucepan. Add remaining corn, broth and dry milk powder. Bring to boil over medium heat, stirring often being careful it doesn't burn on the bottom of the saucepan. Add salt and pepper. Serve hot or chill for a cold soup.

Garnish soup in bowl with grated fresh pepper if desired.

4 Servings.

The best kind of wrinkles
indicate where smiles have been.

Potato Soup (Instant)

2 tablespoons olive oil
½ cup chopped onion
4 cups milk
1¼ cups potato flakes
¼ teaspoon salt
1/8 teaspoon white pepper

Place the 2 tablespoons olive oil in the saucepan, add the chopped onion (and celery if desired). cook until soft. Add the milk, cook over medium heat until hot, but not boiling. Turn off heat and stir in the potato flakes. Season with the salt and pepper.

4 Servings.

Spicy Pumpkin Soup

2 celery stalks
1 small onion
2 tablespoons olive oil
16 ounce can pumpkin
2 cups milk
1 tablespoon cinnamon
2 teaspoons nutmeg
½ teaspoon salt
2 tablespoons molasses
1½ cups water (about)

Chop celery and onion, sauté in olive oil in soup kettle. Stir in pumpkin, milk, seasonings and molasses. Add water for the right consistency, simmer on low, stirring occasionally for about 30 minutes to 1 hour.

4-6 Servings.

Note: Can put soup in blender if desired.

Wisdom is like a comb
that life gives you
after your hair has fallen out.

Scallop Soup

1 pound fresh or thawed frozen scallops,
1 tablespoon lemon juice
½ teaspoon salt
½ teaspoon paprika
1 tablespoon salad oil
4 cups skim milk
1/8 teaspoon nutmeg
1/8 teaspoon white pepper

Cut scallops into bite size pieces. Put scallops in bowl.

Mix lemon juice, salt and paprika. Add to scallops and stir to coat. Let stand 10-15 minutes. Then sauté in the oil 5 minutes, stirring frequently. Add 3 ¾ cups of the milk, nutmeg and pepper. Heat. Thicken with 2 tablespoons flour mixed with the ¼ cup milk left.

4-5 Servings.

Tomato–Consomme
With Rice Soup

2 cups tomato juice
12 ounce can consommé
1/8 teaspoon white pepper
½ cup instant rice

Mix liquids in saucepan. Add pepper and bring to
a boil. Add rice, cover loosely, and simmer about
5 minutes.

4 Servings.

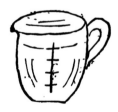

Salmon Chowder

1 cup peeled and cubed potatoes or
     1 cup frozen hash browns or
     16 ounce can whole potatoes
     drained and cubed
1 cup broccoli, cut in bite size pieces
¾ cup celery, cut in bite size pieces
1 small onion, chopped
4 cups milk
½ teaspoon salt
¼ teaspoon white or black pepper
½ teaspoon dill weed
15½ ounce can salmon
3 tablespoons flour mixed in ¼ cup water

Drain salmon, reserving liquid, remove skin and discard, mash bones. Break salmon into bite size pieces and put aside. In large saucepan put potatoes, broccoli, celery, onions, milk, salmon liquid and mashed bones and bring to a boil, lower heat and simmer 15-20 minutes until vegetables are crisp tender. Add seasonings and salmon, heat thoroughly, add flour and water mixture and stir until slightly thickened.

Note: I mash the salmon bones for it is a good source of calcium and add it to the soup.

6-8 Servings.

Seafood Chowder

½ cup chopped celery
1 cup chopped onion
2 teaspoons basil
¼ teaspoon pepper
29 ounce can tomato puree
3 cups broth or water
15 ounce can white beans, drained and rinsed
8 ounces crab or imitation crab, thawed

Place all ingredients, except the crabmeat, in a large soup kettle. Bring to a boil, reduce heat and simmer for 15 minutes.

Add the crab or imitation crab and simmer 3-5 minutes.

8 Servings.

Keep the old as long as it is good,
take the new as soon as it's better.

Cream of Almond Soup

1 cup blanched almonds, toasted (see note)
3 cups turkey broth
1 small onion, coarsely chopped
½ bay leaf
1/8 teaspoon mace
1/8 teaspoon cinnamon
1/8 teaspoon ginger
1 cup milk
2 tablespoons arrowroot or cornstarch

In blender container grind almonds until very fine. Add 1 cup of the broth and onions. Blend until very smooth.

Combine almond mixture, rest of broth and bay leaf in medium saucepan, simmer, covered, 30 minutes. Discard bay leaf. Stir in mace, cinnamon, ginger and milk.

Dissolve 2 tablespoons arrowroot in 2 tablespoons of water. Gradually stir into almond mixture, bring to boiling point, stirring. Ladle into soup bowl; sprinkle lightly with nutmeg if desired. Serve hot or cold.

Note: To toast almonds, spread in ungreased baking pan. Place in 350 degree oven and bake 5- 10 minutes or until almonds are light brown. Stir once or twice. Almonds will continue to brown slightly after removing from oven. 4-6 Servings.

Oatmeal Soup

1 small onion, minced
1 tablespoon olive oil or choice
4 cups vegetable broth
1/3 cup oatmeal
ground pepper, to taste

Cook onion in olive oil until soft and translucent in saucepan. Pour in broth, add oatmeal. Simmer, uncovered about 30 minutes.

2-4 Servings.

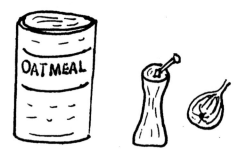

New England Fish Chowder

1 tablespoon olive oil
¾ cup chopped onion
1 clove garlic, crushed or
    ¼ teaspoon garlic powder or
    ½ teaspoon garlic puree
1 bay leaf
1 sprig parsley, cut up or 2 teaspoons dry parsley
1½ cups water
½ teaspoon thyme
¼ salt
1/16 teaspoon white pepper
2 cups skim milk or broth
1 pound frozen cod fillets, partially thawed and cut into 1 inch cubes

Heat oil in saucepan, sauté onions and garlic for a few minutes. Add all other ingredients. Simmer for 45 minutes.

Remove bay leaf, garlic clove and parsley sprig if using.

Can thicken the soup with 2 tablespoons flour mixed with some of the milk.

4 Servings

Cream of Blueberry Soup

1 cup water
12 ounce package frozen blueberries or
    1 pint blueberries
1/3 cup frozen unsweetened pineapple juice
    concentrate
½ teaspoon cinnamon
1½ cups plain yogurt

In a 1½ quart saucepan, bring water to boiling; add blueberries, pineapple concentrate and cinnamon. Boil for 3 minutes. Reduce heat and simmer 10 minutes. Cool.

In blender combine the cooled blueberry mixture with yogurt and blend until smooth.

Serve garnished with a dollop of plain yogurt and a few blueberries.

4 Servings

There are only two kinds of drivers:
the timid mice who drive slower than I do,
and the raving lunatics who drive faster.

Blueberry Soup

1/3 cup unsweetened pineapple juice concentrate
½ cup water
1 teaspoon fresh lemon juice
½ teaspoon vanilla
12 ounce package frozen unsweetened
     blueberries, thawed or 3 cups
     fresh blueberries

Combine pineapple juice concentrate, water, lemon juice and vanilla in blender, add blueberries, puree until smooth.

Serve cold.

Garnish with a dollop of sour cream or yogurt.

4 Servings.

Happiness is a way station
between
too little and too much.

Strawberry Soup

16 ounce package unsweetened frozen
    strawberries, partially thawed or
    1 quart strawberries washed and hulled.
12 ounce can evaporated skim milk
1/3 cup frozen unsweetened pineapple
    juice concentrate
1/8 teaspoon ginger

In blender container puree until smooth, strawberries, milk, pineapple concentrate and ginger.

Garnish with sliced strawberries if desired.

Note: Can add ¼ cup rum if desired.

4-6 Servings

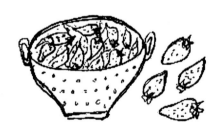

Apple Soup

1 pound tart cooking apples, peeled, cored
    and sliced
3 cups water
2 inch strip of lemon peel
1 tablespoon lemon juice
½ cup frozen unsweetened apple juice concentrate
½ teaspoon cinnamon
¼ teaspoon nutmeg
sour cream

Place all ingredients, except sour cream, in a saucepan (not aluminum) cover, and simmer about 15-20 minutes until apples are mushy. Puree in a blender.

Serve hot or cold with a dollop of sour cream if you like.

4 Servings.

The older we get,
the better we were.

Cherry Soup

12 ounce or 16 ounce package frozen
    bing cherries or dark cherries or
    2 pounds ripe bing cherries pitted
3 cups water
½ cup frozen unsweetened apple juice concentrate
1 stick cinnamon
2 tablespoons lemon juice
1 strip lemon peel
2 tablespoons cornstarch or
    arrowroot dissolved in
    2 tablespoons of water

Simmer cherries, water, apple concentrate, cinnamon stick, lemon juice and lemon peel 10 minutes. Add cornstarch and water mixture and simmer few minutes more. Remove cinnamon stick and lemon strip.

Garnish with dollop of yogurt or sour cream if desired.

Can serve hot or cold.

4 Servings.

Peach Soup

16 ounce package frozen peaches, partially
     thawed or 4 large ripe peaches,
     peeled and quartered
1/3 cup frozen unsweetened pineapple
     juice concentrate
1/8 teaspoon cinnamon
1/8 teaspoon nutmeg
½ teaspoon vanilla
12 ounce can evaporated skim milk

Combine all ingredients in blender or food processor until smooth.

Chill in refrigerator, stir well, serve cold. Or
serve after blending.

Sprinkle lightly with nutmeg if desired.

5 Servings.

A person is not rewarded for having brain
only for using them.

Plum Soup

4 cups water
1/3 cup frozen unsweetened pineapple
    juice concentrate
1½ pounds purple plums, small, halved and pitted
2 inch strip of lemon peel
1 inch cinnamon stick
1 tablespoon arrowroot dissolved in
        1 tablespoon cold water
½ cup unsweetened apple juice or Port wine
1 cup plain yogurt

In stainless steel or enameled saucepan combine water, pineapple concentrate and bring to a boil. Add the 1½ pounds purple plums halved and pitted, lemon peel and cinnamon stick, cook covered, over moderate heat. Stir occasionally for 30 minutes or until plums are very soft.
Discard the lemon peel and cinnamon stick.

Puree the mixture in a blender or food processor. Put back into saucepan, bring puree to a boil, stir in arrowroot mixture and cook about 5 minutes or until slightly thickened.

Remove pan from heat and stir in the apple juice or port wine. Pour into bowl, chill mixture about 3 hours.

(Continued on next page)

In small bowl mix 1 cup of the plum mixture into 1 cup plain yogurt. Stir the mixture into remaining plum mixture.

Garnish with a dollop of yogurt sprinkled with cinnamon.

Note: Can serve hot and do not add the yogurt. The yogurt is optional.

4-6 Servings.

Ability is a wonderful thing,
but its value is greatly enhanced by
dependability.

Cranberry Soup

12 ounce package fresh cranberries
1 large cinnamon stick
2 cups water
2/3 cup unsweetened pineapple juice concentrate
½ teaspoon vanilla extract
12 ounces evaporated skim milk or
      fat free plain yogurt

Place cranberries and cinnamon stick in large saucepan. Add water, bring to a boil at medium heat, reduce heat and simmer, covered, until cranberries are very tender and begin to fall apart, about 15 minutes. Remove cinnamon stick. Pour berries in a blender or food processor. Puree and then rub threw a strainer. Discard solids. Place cranberry mixture, pineapple juice concentrate, vanilla and evaporated milk in saucepan and reheat just under a boil. Can be served hot or cold.

When serving, top with a tablespoon of plain yogurt and a dash of nutmeg.

Note: Can be made without the evaporated milk or yogurt.

4 Servings.

Melon – Lime Soup

3 cups seeded, peeled and cubed honey dew melon, chilled
¼ cup frozen pineapple juice concentrate
1 tablespoon lime juice
8 ounce carton fat free plain yogurt or sour cream

In blender, place melon cubes, pineapple concentrate and lime juice, blend until smooth. Add the yogurt or sour cream and blend until smooth.

Garnish each serving with lime peel curls or a lime slice.

4 Servings.

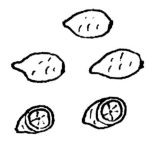

Swedish Fruit Soup

1/2 package (4 ounces) prunes
1/2 package (4 ounces) peaches
1/2 package (4 ounces) apricots
1/2 package (7-1/2 ounces) raisins,
     dark &/or light
2 cups apple juice (optional)

Put prunes, peaches, apricots and raisins in a kettle, cover with water and cook slowly until fruit is tender, about 1-1/2 hours. Add more water if needed. Add apple juice and simmer 5-10 minutes more. Serve either hot or cold.

Note: can substitute a package of mixed fruit for some of the fruit.

8 Servings.

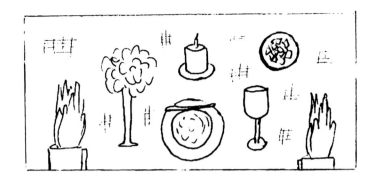

Chapter 5

Main Dishes

Salmon Loaf

15 ½ ounce can salmon
1 cup oatmeal
¼ cup milk
2 eggs, beaten or egg substitute
2 tablespoons lemon juice
2 tablespoons finely chopped onion
2 tablespoons chopped fresh parsley or
      1 tablespoon dried parsley flakes
¼ teaspoon salt
1/8 teaspoon pepper

Spray an 8x4 inch loaf pan

Drain salmon. Remove skin and discard, mash bones. Flake the salmon in a medium size bowl, combine salmon and remaining ingredients, mix just until blended .

Turn into loaf pan. Bake in a 350 degrees oven for 40-45 minutes.

6-8 Servings.

Pork and Rice Casserole

1 pound pork, cooked and cubed
1 large onion, chopped
¾ cup uncooked rice
1¾ cups broth

Mix ingredients in casserole dish.

Bake, covered, in 350 degrees oven for 1½ hours.
Remove cover last 30 minutes of baking.

Note: Can use leftover cooked beef or other leftover meat.

4-6 Servings.

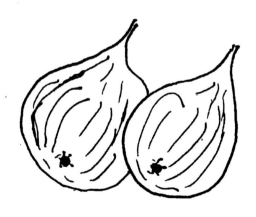

Speedy Leftover Beef & Vegetables

10 ounce package frozen mixed vegetables
½ cup sliced onions
¼ cup water
¾ cup tomato juice
1 cup cooked roast beef, sliced
1 tablespoon light soy sauce
1/8 teaspoon ground ginger

Combine vegetables and water in a non-stick skillet. Cover and simmer 2 minutes. Stir in remaining ingredients. Cook and stir until liquid evaporates to a thick glaze, about 3-4 minutes.

2-3 Servings.

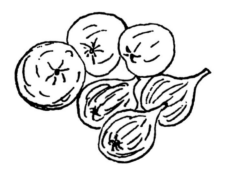

Lentil Loaf

2 cups cooked lentils
½ cup chopped walnuts
1 egg or egg substitute
1 can fat free evaporated milk
½ teaspoon dried basil
½ teaspoon dried thyme
½ teaspoon salt
2 cups crushed cereal flakes
¼ cup vegetable oil

Mix all ingredients well. Place in loaf pan and bake in 350 degrees oven for 45 minutes.

4-6 Servings.

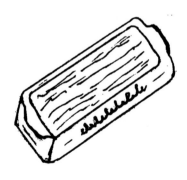

Meat Loaf

1½ pounds lean ground beef
1 cup oatmeal
2 eggs, beaten or egg substitute
1 cup fat free milk or tomato juice
½ teaspoon salt
¼ teaspoon pepper
1 tablespoon prepared mustard
½ teaspoon onion powder

Combine. Put in vegetable sprayed loaf pan.

Bake in 375 degrees oven for 1 hour.

Note: For burgers reduce milk ½ cup.

6-8 Servings.

Do the very best you can today
And tomorrow you can do better.

Meat Loaf with Onion Soup

2 pounds lean ground beef
1 envelope onion soup mix
1½ cups fresh bread crumbs
2 eggs, beaten or egg substitute
¾ cup water
1/3 cup tomato sauce

In large bowl, combine all ingredients.

In baking pan, shape mixture into a loaf .

Bake in 350 degrees oven for 1 hour or until done.

6-8 Servings.

The really happy person is the one who can enjoy the scenery, even when they've taken a detour.

Stir Fry

Sauce:
1 tablespoon cornstarch or arrowroot
3 tablespoons light soy sauce
1 cup water

Combine sauce ingredients. Set aside.

1 pound chicken, turkey or beef cut into
       1 x ½ inch pieces
16 ounces broccoli, chopped
1 small onion, chopped or sliced
2 teaspoons vegetable oil
¼ teaspoon red pepper flakes

Add 1 teaspoon oil to nonstick skillet, heat and add meat and stir fry about 3-5 minutes, remove from pan. Add the other 1 teaspoon oil to skillet and add the chopped vegetables and onions, stir fry 3-5 minutes. Add the red pepper flakes. Stir in sauce ingredients and cook until sauce thickens.

Stir in meat and heat through.

Serve over rice or noodles.

4 Servings.

Turkey Stir Fry

1 pound turkey breasts, cut into 1 x ½ inch pieces
2 teaspoons olive oil or canola oil
16 ounce package frozen mixed vegetables
2 tablespoons Teriyaki sauce

Sauté breasts in 1 teaspoon olive oil in nonstick skillet 3-5 minutes. Remove from skillet. Add the other teaspoon oil and sauté vegetables 3-5 minutes. Put meat back in skillet and add the Teriyaki sauce, heat through.

4 Servings.

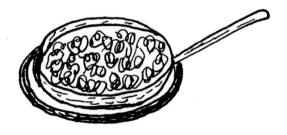

Skillet Turkey and Bows

¾ pound ground turkey
1 medium onion, chopped
¼ teaspoon garlic powder
14½ ounce can stewed tomatoes
¼ cup light soy sauce
1¼ teaspoons dried basil, crumbled
2 ½ cups, uncooked, bow tie macaroni
8 ounces frozen cut green beans

Cook turkey with onion and garlic powder in large nonstick skillet (with cover) over medium heat, breaking up turkey. Stir in tomatoes, soy sauce, basil and 1¼ cups water; cover and bring to a boil. Stir in macaroni; cover and return to boil. Reduce heat and simmer 15 minutes, stirring once. Stir in green beans; cover and return to boil. Reduce heat and simmer 10-12 minutes longer or until macaroni and beans are tender, stirring occasionally.

4 Servings.

Pleasant words are as honeycomb.
sweet to the soul and health to the body

Pumpkin Chili

1 pound lean ground beef
16 ounce can pumpkin
2 teaspoons chili powder
1 teaspoon onion powder
½ teaspoon salt
¼ teaspoon pepper
32 ounce jar tomatoes
16 ounce can red beans

Brown ground beef, add pumpkin, chili powder, onion powder, salt, pepper and tomatoes. Simmer 30 minutes, add red beans and simmer until beans are heated.

5-6 Servings.

Life is full of shadows,
but the sunshine makes them all.

Three Bean Chili

16 ounce can navy beans
16 ounce can pinto beans
16 ounce can red beans
10½ ounce can condensed onion soup,
      do not dilute
1 teaspoon ginger
1 teaspoon cumin
1 tablespoon prepared hot mustard
¼ cup molasses

In a large kettle, put beans and onion soup.
Add remaining ingredients, bring to a boil and
simmer 45 minutes to 1 hour, stirring occasionally.

6-8 Servings.

*Blessed is s/he whose daily tasks are a labor of
love, for willing hands and happy heart translate
duty into privilege, and labor becomes service.*

Lamb with Cabbage

8-12 ounces leftover cooked lamb, trimmed
     and cut into 1 inch pieces
1½ cups turkey broth
1 cup water
½ bay leaf
16 ounce package cabbage and carrot coleslaw
1 cup instant mashed potatoes

Bring the broth, water and bay leaf to a boil, add the coleslaw and lamb, simmer, covered for 20 minutes. Add the mashed potato flakes and stir in, reheat a few minutes or until hot.

Remove bay leaf and serve.

4-6 Servings.

*If you see someone who needs a smile,
give them one of yours.*

Stir Fry Chicken

2 skinless, boneless, chicken breasts,
    cut in thin strips
16 ounce package Oriental blend frozen
    vegetables, thawed
1½ cups chicken broth
1½ tablespoons cornstarch or arrowroot
3 tablespoons soy sauce
3 tablespoons dry red wine or white wine or
    vermouth
8 ounce can sliced water chestnuts
hot cooked rice

Spray a non-stick skillet with vegetable oil, heat and sauté chicken, stirring constantly, 5-10 minutes until tender. Remove chicken.

Add thawed frozen vegetables and ½ of the chicken broth. Cook uncovered 5 minutes or until vegetables are slightly crisp. Meanwhile combine cornstarch, soy sauce, wine and remaining broth. Pour over vegetables. Cook and stir until sauce thickens. Add chicken and chestnuts. Heat through. Serve with rice.

4 Servings.

Quick & Easy Skillet Chicken

1 envelope onion soup mix (about 1¼ ounces)
¾ cup water
1 pound boneless and skinless chicken or
      turkey breast, cut into thin stripes
16 ounce package frozen mixed vegetables,
      thawed
hot cooked rice

In large skillet blend onion soup mix with water. Bring to a boil; stir in chicken or turkey, cook 2-3 minutes, then stir in vegetables. Cook uncovered, stirring frequently 5 minutes or until chicken or turkey is done.

Serve over hot rice.

4-5 Servings.

*Blessed is s/he who mends stockings and toys and
broken hearts,
for understanding is balm to humanity*

Turkey – Celery Dish

1 medium onion, chopped
1½ cups turkey or chicken broth
3 cups sliced celery
1 tablespoon light soy sauce
4 ounce jar sliced mushrooms, drained
2 cups cooked chicken or turkey, cut up
2 tablespoons cornstarch or arrowroot

In 3 quart saucepan put onions, broth, celery
and soy sauce, bring to a boil, cover and simmer
15-20 minutes, until celery and onions are crisp
tender.

Add the mushrooms and turkey, heat to boiling.

Mix the cornstarch with a little water, stir into
mixture, stirring until smooth. Put in serving dish.

Garnish with parsley sprigs.

6 Servings

Tuna Patties

½ cup mashed potato flakes
1 teaspoon parsley flakes
1 teaspoon onion flakes or powder
½ teaspoon dry mustard
½ cup milk
2 - 6 ½ ounce cans tuna, drained
2 eggs

In medium bowl, combine all ingredients.

Spray a non-stick skillet with vegetable oil.

Using a 1/3 cup size measuring cup scoop into heated skillet, spreading to size desired; repeat with remaining mixture. Fry patties until deep golden brown on both sides.

6 Servings.

*The happiest people don't necessarily HAVE
the best of everything;
they must MAKE the best of everything.*

Crustless Smoked Salmon Quiche

15½ ounce can salmon
1 teaspoon lemon juice
6 ounces shredded mozzarella or Swiss cheese
½ teaspoon dill weed
¾ cup milk (about)
4 eggs
½ teaspoon liquid smoke
¼ teaspoon salt
1/8 teaspoon pepper
½ cup biscuit
paprika

Drain salmon, saving juice, remove any skin and discard, mash bones. Break up salmon and place in medium bowl, along with the mashed bones, toss with lemon juice, set aside.

Add to salmon juice enough milk to make 1 cup. Add to salmon, cheese and dill weed until blended. Transfer to well sprayed vegetable oiled quiche or 9 inch pie plate.

In small bowl, mix milk mixture, eggs, liquid smoke, salt, pepper and biscuit, mix until well blended. Pour over salmon mixture. Lightly sprinkle with paprika.

Bake in 350 degrees oven 45 minutes or until knife inserted in center comes out clean. Cool 10 minutes.

4 – 6 Servings.

No Crust Quiche

10 ounces frozen broccoli spears
1 small onion, chopped
1 cup shredded mozzarella or other low fat cheese
1½ cups milk
4 eggs or egg substitute
½ teaspoon salt
1/8 teaspoon pepper
¾ cup biscuit mix

Preheat oven to 400 degrees. Spray quiche pan or 8 or 9 inch cake pan well. Cut broccoli spears into bite size pieces, put in greased pan, put onions over broccoli, then grated cheese.

Beat together the remaining ingredients until smooth, pour over vegetables and cheese.

Bake 35-40 minutes. Let stand 5 minutes before serving.

This dish can be prepared ahead and refrigerated. To reheat, cover with foil and bake in 350 degrees oven for 15-20 minutes.

4 – 6 Servings.

Zucchini Quiche Dish
(No crust or cheese)

3 cups zucchini (about 12 ounces) unpeeled and
    thinly sliced
½ cup onion, chopped or sliced
¼ teaspoon basil
¼ teaspoon oregano
¼ teaspoon salt
1/8 teaspoon pepper
6 eggs, beaten or egg substitute
2 tablespoons nonfat dry milk

Layer zucchini and onions in a well sprayed with
vegetable oil a 10 inch glass pie plate or quiche
dish.

Mix basil, oregano, salt and pepper and sprinkle
over vegetables.

Beat eggs or egg substitute, add dry milk. Pour
over zucchini mixture in pie plate.

Bake in 350 degree oven for about 35 minutes.

4-6 Servings.

Note: Can mix all ingredients in large bowl and
pour mixture into prepared dish. (Mixing milk
into eggs before adding to mixture).

Turkey Chop Suey

4 cups diced cooked turkey, or other cooked meat
4 large stalks celery, cut into ½ inch slices
4 medium onions, chopped
3 ounce jar sliced mushrooms, drained
3 cups water
3 tablespoons soy sauce
2 – 16 ounce cans chop suey vegetables

In saucepan combine first 6 ingredients. Simmer for 35-45 minutes or until celery is tender. Stir in the chop suey vegetables, and heat thoroughly.

Thicken with 3 tablespoons cornstarch mixed with 4 tablespoons water.

Chop suey can be served over hot cooked rice and topped with Chinese noodles.

6 Servings.

Salmon Quiche

12 ounces cooked salmon, flaked
1 cup grated mozzarella cheese
1 cup fat free milk
4 large eggs, lightly beaten or egg substitute
2 tablespoons flour
1 teaspoon dill weed
1 tablespoon lemon juice
½ teaspoon salt
¼ teaspoon pepper

Put the cooked flaked salmon in a vegetable
sprayed 10 inch pie plate or quiche dish, sprinkle
the cheese over the salmon.

In a bowl combine the milk, eggs, flour, dill
weed, lemon juice, salt and pepper, blend well.
Pour mixture over the cheese and bake in a
preheated 375 degree oven for 40 minutes.
Let stand 10 minutes before serving.

6 Servings.

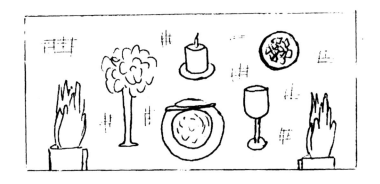

Chapter 6

Meats, Poultry, Fish

Poached Turkey Breast & Homemade Turkey Broth

1 whole turkey breast on the bone (5½ pounds)
2 carrots
2 stalks celery
2 onions, halved
1 bay leaf
½ teaspoon dried thyme, crumbled
2 cans reduced sodium chicken broth or
      3½ cups broth of choice

Place the turkey breast in a Dutch oven. Add the carrots, celery, onions, bay leaf, thyme and the broth. Add enough water to cover. Bring to boiling, lower heat to simmering, cover, and cook for 1¼ hours or until inner temperature of the turkey registers 160 degree.

Remove the turkey and let stand until cool enough to handle. Remove the skin from the turkey and discard. Remove the breast meat from the bone.

Remove the vegetables from the broth with a slotted spoon and discard.

Strain the broth if needed and discard the solids. Chill the broth and discard the fat from the top.

Can make gravy from the broth. 6 Servings.

Chicken Breast with Rice

1 cup uncooked rice
14 ounce can chicken broth
¾ cup water
½ teaspoon dill weed
1 tablespoon parsley flakes.
½ teaspoon dried oregano
1/8 teaspoon pepper
6 chicken breasts
paprika

Place rice, broth, water, dill weed, parsley flakes and oregano in a vegetable sprayed shallow baking pan (9x13). Place chicken breasts on top of rice mixture. Sprinkle breasts lightly with paprika and pepper. Cover pan with aluminum foil.

Bake in 325 degrees oven for 1½ - 2 hours.

4-6 Servings.

Baked Pork Chops

4 loin pork chops cut ½ - ¾ inch thick
1 medium yellow onion, sliced or chopped
¾ cup beef broth
1 bay leaf
1 cup fat free sour cream

Cut fat from chops, discard fat. Spray a nonstick skillet with vegetable oil, heat pan and brown chops 5 minutes on each side over moderate heat.

Put chops in a 9x12 inch baking pan or large casserole dish, sprinkle lightly with salt and pepper. Add broth, onion and bay leaf to pan, simmer a few minutes, pour over chops in baking dish, cover with aluminum foil.

Put in preheated 350 degrees oven 50-60 minutes or until well done.

Transfer chops to serving dish.

Pour juices into a saucepan and add sour cream, heat about 1 minute, do not boil. Pour sauce over meat and serve.

Note: Can add 4 ounce jar sliced mushrooms, drained, to sour cream mixture if desired.

3-4 Servings.

Easy Brisket

1 cup catsup or tomato sauce
1 cup ginger ale
1 envelope onion soup mix (about 1¼ ounces)
2½ - 3 pounds brisket of beef, trimmed
¼ cup dry red wine
Hot rice

Combine catsup or tomato sauce, ginger ale and soup mix in Dutch oven. Add brisket, turning several times to coat all sides with sauce. Bring to boil over medium heat, reduce heat, add wine, cover and simmer until tender, about 2 to 4 hours, adding water if necessary to keep meat moist.

Transfer meat to cutting board and slice thinly. Return to sauce and heat through.

Serve over rice.

6-8 Servings.

Beef Tenderloin Tips

3-4 pounds tenderloin tips or boneless beef
      chuck, cut into 1 inch pieces
2 medium onions, diced or cut into slices
6 ounce jar button mushrooms, drained
¼ cup flour
1 cup dry red wine
2 cans (10½ ounces) French onion soup
2 soup cans water
salt and pepper

In large non-stick skillet, sprayed with vegetable oil and heated, sauté beef pieces until brown on all sides, add onions, sauté until onions are wilted. Sprinkle with flour, stir in red wine, onion soup, water and mushrooms. Stir to blend. Cover and simmer 1½ -2 hours, stirring occasionally or put in 325 degrees oven.

Season to taste with salt and pepper if you like.

Note: Tenderloin tips may take only 50-60 minutes.

6 Servings.

Salmon Steaks

2 tablespoons olive oil
2 cups chopped onions
4 salmon fillets (6 ounces each) skinned
1/3 cup reduced sodium soy sauce

Heat oil in large nonstick skillet over medium heat, add onions, cook stirring occasionally, until translucent, about 5 minutes.

Place salmon fillets over onions in skillet, pour on soy sauce. Cover and simmer over low heat until salmon is opaque in center, 10-12 minutes.

Put salmon on serving platter. Continue cooking onions and soy sauce, uncovered, until slightly thickened, 2–3 minutes.

Pour over salmon and serve.

4 Servings.

There are two ways of spreading light --
to be the candle, or the mirror that reflects it.

Herb Baked Fish

1 pound frozen haddock, halibut or cod
1 tablespoon olive oil
½ teaspoon salt
½ teaspoon garlic powder
¼ teaspoon oregano
¼ teaspoon thyme
1/16 teaspoon pepper
1 small bay leaf
½ cup thinly sliced onion, separated into rings
½ cup evaporated skim milk

Place frozen fish in a 10x6x1½ inches baking dish. Rub oil over fish and sprinkle with seasonings. Add bay leaf. Arrange onion rings over fish and pour milk in dish.

Bake, uncovered in 350 degrees oven about 30-40 minutes.

Garnish with lemon slices and parsley.

4 Servings.

Joy is not in things;

Baked Scallops

1½ pounds scallops, if using frozen, thaw
½ teaspoon salt
1/8 teaspoon pepper
1 tablespoon lemon juice
1 cup fat-free cream sauce
paprika
cooked rice or noodles, optional

Prepare scallops, season with the salt, pepper and lemon juice, let marinade while preparing cream sauce.

Cover bottom of vegetable sprayed baking dish with a little of the sauce. Repeat with scallops and sauce. Sprinkle lightly with paprika.

Bake 15-20 minutes, depending on the size of the scallops, in a 350 degree oven.

Can be served over rice or noodles.

4-6 Servings.

Note: Fat-free cream sauce recipe is on pg. 92.

Fish-Vegetable Dish

2 pounds cod or haddock fillets
2 cups milk
2 bay leaves
8 ounces frozen peas and diced carrots
2 tablespoons cornstarch or arrowroot
¼ teaspoon salt
1/16 teaspoon white pepper

Place fish in pan, add the milk and bay leaves. Bring to a boil, cover and simmer 5-7 minutes. Using a slotted spoon remove the fish from the pan, flake fish with 2 forks into bite size pieces. Put aside.

Put the peas and carrots into the pan, bring back to a boil and simmer, covered, and cook 5-7 minutes.

Mix the cornstarch or arrowroot with a little water and add to the vegetable mixture in pan and cook until slightly thickened; add the flaked fish. Discard the bay leaf and season to taste with the salt and pepper. Put in serving dish

Note: Can be served over cooked noodles or rice.

4 Servings.

Dinner Fillets

½ lemon, thinly sliced
1 onion, thinly sliced
2 pounds fish, mackerel, cod or haddock,
        cut into serving size
½ teaspoon salt
¼ teaspoon white pepper
paprika
¾ cup chicken, turkey or vegetable broth

Place lemon slices in layer in 9x13 inch baking dish, put onion slice over lemon. Place fish on onion, sprinkle with salt, pepper and paprika.
Pour broth around fillets in dish.

Bake in 400 degrees oven for 12 minutes or until fish flakes easily with fork. Remove fish to serving platter. Top with lemon and onion slice.
Garnish with parsley sprigs.

4-6 Servings.

Prepared it in the microwave 10 minutes.

The best things in life
Aren't things.

195

Baked Fish

1 pound fish fillets, cod, haddock or red snapper
1/3 cup fat free mayonnaise
½ teaspoon dill weed
½ teaspoon onion powder
¼ teaspoon garlic powder
½ cup crushed saltine crackers

Spray a 9x13 inch baking dish with vegetable oil. Place fish in dish.

Combine mayonnaise and seasonings, spread over fish. Top with crumbs.

Bake in 350 degrees oven for 20-30 minutes or until fish flakes easily.

4 Servings.

We are what we have learned from the past,
what we experience today,
and what we dream for tomorrow.

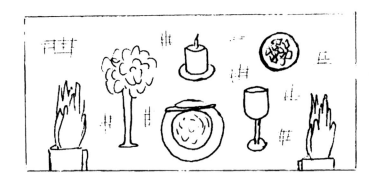

Chapter 7

Pasta, Rice

Fettuccini Alfredo

1 cup evaporated skim milk
1 teaspoon oil
¼ cup fat free cream cheese
8 ounces fettuccini
1/8 teaspoon white pepper
½ cup Parmesan cheese, grated

In large saucepan, combine milk and oil. Cook over medium heat until milk simmers. Add cream cheese, cook and stir until cream cheese melts and mixture is smooth, add pepper, cover and remove from heat.

Meanwhile cook fettuccini according to package directions, drain. Add fettuccini to milk mixture in pan, cook over low heat tossing until well coated, about 1 minute. Add Parmesan cheese, toss lightly to combine. Remove from heat. Cover and let stand 1-2 minutes.

When serving sprinkle with more Parmesan cheese if desired.

Note: Can use other pasta shapes.

4-6 Servings.

Pasta with Garlic and Oil

9 ounce package noodles or fettuccini
¼ cup olive oil
1 clove garlic or ½ teaspoon garlic puree
1 tablespoon dried parsley or
      2 tablespoons fresh parsley
½ teaspoon salt or to taste
1/8 teaspoon white pepper or to taste
Parmesan cheese, grated

Cook the pasta according to package directions.

Meanwhile make the sauce. Heat the oil, garlic, parsley, salt and pepper in a large sauce pan.

Drain the pasta and add to the sauce in the sauce-pan, toss to coat well.

Put in a dish and serve with Parmesan cheese.

4-6 Servings.

Salmon Pasta

1 onion, thinly sliced
6 ounce jar sliced mushrooms
4 cups cooked linguine
¼ cup Parmesan cheese, grated
¼ cup dry white wine or apple juice
¼ cup fat free mayonnaise
¼ cup fat free plain yogurt
¼ teaspoon nutmeg
15½ ounce can salmon or 2 cups cooked salmon
½ teaspoon dill weed

Spray a large non-stick skillet, well, with vegetable oil. Brown onions over medium heat, mix in cooked linguine, mushrooms and liquid, Parmesan cheese, wine, mayonnaise, yogurt and nutmeg, lower heat to low and heat until pasta is lightly coated, add salmon, cover and leave over low heat until heated through.

Sprinkle with dill weed just before serving.

8 Servings.

Cavatini

3 cups uncooked pasta, varied shapes
4 ounce jar button mushrooms
¼ cup sliced green olives
¼ cup sliced black olives
1 medium onion, chopped
15½ ounce jar spaghetti sauce
8 ounces tomato sauce
1 cup shredded cheese, Mexican style is good
8 ounces shredded Mozzarella cheese

In large saucepan cook pasta, boil under tender. Drain.

Meanwhile put remaining ingredients, except Mozzarella cheese, in large bowl and mix well. Add cooked pasta and mix well.

Place in large casserole dish or 9x13 inch pan. Bake covered with foil in 350 degrees oven until bubbly, about 35-40 minutes.

Remove from oven, sprinkle with the Mozzarella cheese. Return to oven and bake until cheese melts.

6-8 Servings.

Spinach Lasagna

15 ounces ricotta cheese
¼ cup Parmesan cheese
1 egg or egg substitute
¼ teaspoon pepper
10 ounce package frozen chopped spinach,
      thawed and drained or squeezed
26 ounce jar spaghetti sauce
8 lasagna noodles, uncooked
6 ounces Mozzarella cheese, grated

Stir together ricotta cheese, Parmesan cheese, egg substitute, pepper and drained spinach.

Spread 1 cup spaghetti sauce in a 13x9x2 inch baking dish. Top with half the noodles, half the spinach mixture, half the remaining sauce. Repeat layers, ending with sauce. Cover with aluminum foil, refrigerate overnight.

Set out about 30 minutes before baking.

Bake, covered, for 50-55 minutes. Remove cover, sprinkle with mozzarella cheese, bake 5 minutes more. Let set 10 minutes before serving.

8 Servings.

Fettuccini with Olive Sauce

12 ounce package Fettuccini noodles
¼ cup olive or salad oil
6 ounce can sliced ripe olives, drained
3 ounce jar pimento-stuffed green olives,
     drained and sliced
small bunch parsley, stems removed, chopped
1 teaspoon dried oregano leaves, crushed
½ teaspoon crushed red pepper
½ cup grated Parmesan cheese

In saucepot prepare fettuccini as label directs, drain. Return fettuccini to pot; keep warm.

Meanwhile in 2 quart saucepan, over medium heat, in hot oil, stir in ripe olives, pimento stuffed olives, parsley, oregano, red pepper and ½ cup water, heat just to boiling, stirring mixture occasionally.

Stir olive mixture into fettuccini in saucepot . Add Parmesan cheese, toss until well mixed

4-6 Servings.

Linguine with Parsley Pesto Sauce

1 pound linguine or spaghetti
1 cup parsley sprigs, stems removed
1 clove garlic
1 tablespoon dried basil
½ cup olive or salad oil
¼ cup water
½ cup grated Parmesan cheese
dash pepper

Cook linguine according to package directions, stirring occasionally, until tender. Drain in colander.

While linguine is cooking, combine parsley, garlic, basil, oil and water in blender. Blend until smooth. Gradually add Parmesan cheese until well mixed. Season to taste with salt and pepper.

Toss linguine with sauce and serve. Can lightly sprinkle with more Parmesan cheese if you like.

4 – 6 Servings.

People usually quarrel
because they cannot argue.

Spaghetti with
Broccoli Pesto Sauce

16 ounces spaghetti
16 ounce package frozen chopped broccoli
1 cup vegetable or turkey or chicken broth
¼ cup grated Parmesan cheese
2 tablespoons olive oil
1 garlic clove
¼ teaspoon salt
grated ground black pepper

In saucepan, prepare pasta in salted boiling water as label directs.
Meanwhile in saucepan steam broccoli as label directs.

In food processor, with knife blade attached, blend cooked broccoli, broth, Parmesan cheese, olive oil, garlic and salt until smooth, stopping processor occasionally to scrape down side.

Drain pasta, toss with broccoli pesto.
Sprinkle with ground black pepper.

4 Servings.

Cold Peanut Butter Noodles

3 tablespoons soy sauce
2 tablespoons rice vinegar or white wine vinegar
½ teaspoon dried hot pepper flakes
½ cup creamy peanut butter
1 tablespoon sesame or olive oil
¼ teaspoon ginger
¾ cup broth
1 pound linguine
chopped peanuts for garnish, optional

In saucepan combine the soy sauce, vinegar, red pepper flakes, peanut butter, oil, ginger and the broth, simmer, stirring until thickened and smooth, let it cool slightly.

Meanwhile in kettle of boiling salted water, cook the noodles until they are al dente, drain them in a colander and rinse under cold water.

Drain the noodles well, transfer them to a bowl and toss them with the sauce.

Serve the noodles at room temperature and garnish with the chopped peanuts.

4-6 Servings

Parsley Rice Squares

3 cups cooked rice
½ cup chopped parsley
½ cup low fat shredded cheese
¼ cup chopped onion
½ teaspoon salt
3 beaten eggs or egg substitute
1½ cups milk

Mix rice, parsley, cheese, onion and seasoning.

Combine eggs and milk, add to rice mixture and mix thoroughly. Pour into vegetable sprayed 10x6x1½ inch baking dish.

Bake in 325 degrees oven for 40 minutes or just until set. Cut into squares.

6-8 Servings.

Blessed is s/he who opens the door to welcome both stranger and friends, for gracious hospitality is a best of love.

Tuna Rice Special

1 cup rice
2½ cups broth
½ teaspoon salt
1/8 teaspoon pepper
1 cup chopped celery
¼ cup sliced stuffed olives
3 tablespoons chopped green pepper
4 ounce bottle or can sliced mushrooms
6½ ounce can tuna

Put rice, broth and seasonings in a 3 quart saucepan. Add celery, olives, green pepper, mushrooms and tuna. Cover and bring to a boil. Simmer for 20 minutes.

Put in serving dish. Garnish with green pepper rings if desired.

6-8 Servings.

Seconds count,
especially when dieting!

Tuna Squares

2 - 6 ½ ounce cans tuna
1 cup cooked rice
1 cup oatmeal
½ teaspoon poultry seasoning
1/3 cup diced celery
4 eggs, beaten or egg substitute
2 cups broth

Combine all ingredients and put in a 9x9 inch sprayed baking dish.

Bake in a 350 degrees oven for 1 hour.

Cut into squares.

Serve with a low fat sauce if desired.

6 - 9 Servings.

God mat og gode venner går godt sammen

(Good food and good friends go well together.)

Brown Rice

1 onion, chopped
1½ tablespoons parsley, chopped
1 teaspoon thyme
1 teaspoon dill
1 teaspoon basil
1 teaspoon oregano
2 tablespoons olive oil
2 1/3 cups broth
1 cup brown rice

In heavy saucepan sauté the onion, parsley, thyme, dill, basil and oregano in the oil over moderately high heat until the onion is soft. Stir in the brown rice and sauté for 3 minutes. Add broth, simmer, covered for 45-50 minutes or until liquid is absorbed and the rice is tender.

Note: Can use dried parsley flakes if desired, about 2 teaspoons.

4-6 Servings.

Smiles are like colds,
they're contagious.

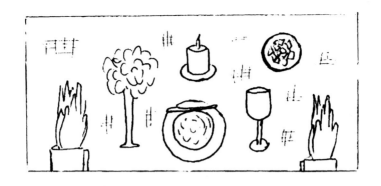

Chapter 8

Sandwiches, Breads

Salmon Burgers

15 ounce can salmon
1 egg or ¼ cup egg substitute
½ teaspoon onion powder or
       ½ cup chopped onions
1 teaspoon dried parsley or
       1 tablespoon fresh parsley
2 teaspoons lemon juice
1 teaspoon Worcestershire sauce or
       teriyaki sauce
½ cup oatmeal
dash pepper

Drain salmon, remove skin and discard, mash bones and flake salmon, combine with all other ingredients. Form into 5-6 patties.

Spray a non-stick skillet with vegetable oil, heat pan and fry patties until golden brown on both sides.

Also good to serve patties with creamed peas.

5-6 Servings

Minds are like parachutes.
They only function when open.

Broccoli Sandwich

8 ounces frozen broccoli
8 slices bread or Italian loaf halved lengthwise
¼ cup fat free mayonnaise
¼ shredded mozzarella cheese

Cook broccoli according to package directions.
Cut broccoli into bite size pieces.

Stir the mayonnaise into broccoli. Spread the broccoli mixture on four bread slices, sprinkle cheese over broccoli mixture. Put remaining bread slices over.

Note: Can add pimento stuffed green olives, sliced, to broccoli mixture if you like.

4 Servings.

If the world seems cold to you,
kindle a fire to warm it.

Eggplant Sandwich

1 eggplant (about 4-6 inches in diameter)
pizza or barbecue sauce
part skim, mozzarella cheese, grated
oregano
whole wheat bread or
    ½ English muffin or bagel

Cut eggplant into ½ inch slices and saute in a non-stick skillet, sprayed with vegetable oil, brown lightly on both sides.

Toast bread or English muffin or bagel.

Put eggplant on toast, top with about 1 teaspoon pizza or barbecue sauce, a little mozzarella cheese and sprinkle lightly with oregano.

Note: Peel the eggplant if the skin is tough, also can put the sandwich in the oven for a few minutes if you would like the cheese melted.

4 Servings.

Life is hard by the yard,
but by the inch it's a cinch.

Cream Cheese Sandwich

4 ounces fat free cream cheese, softened
¼ cup chopped parsley
¼ cup chopped peanuts or other nuts
¼ cup chopped pimento stuffed olives
12 slices whole wheat or rye bread

Cream cheese, add parsley, peanuts and olives. Spread between 6 slices of bread, cover with the other 6 slices.

6 Servings.

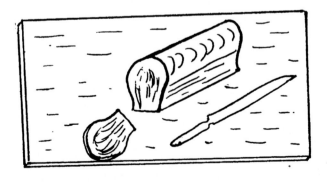

Quick Cream Cheese Sandwich

8 ounces fat free cheese cream, softened
8 slices whole wheat or rye bread

Spread 1 tablespoon cream cheese over the slices of bread. Put one of the following, or your own choice, over 4 slices.

1-Chopped nuts and sliced pimiento stuffed olives.
2-Chopped nuts, raisins, or currents.
3-Chopped figs, dates, raisins or prunes.
4-Peanut butter and raspberry or strawberry jam or choice.
5-Shredded carrots and cabbage or lettuce leaf.
6-Canned sliced beets
7-Pineapple slice
8-Shredded carrots, raisins or currents.

Cover filling with the other four slices of bread, cheese side over the filling. Cut each sandwich diagonally into four pieces.

4 Servings.

Note: Can use a cheese spread in place of the cream cheese.

Pressed Sandwich Loaf

6-8 inch round Italian or sour dough bread
1 tablespoon olive oil
6½ ounce can light tuna in water, drained
2 ounce can flat anchovies in olive oil, optional
7 ounce jar roasted sweet peppers, drained
16 ounce jar mild pepper rings, optional
1 tomato, sliced and peeled

Cut bread in half horizontally. Place bottom half on large plate. Brush both cut sides with olive oil. Spoon tuna evenly over bread on plate, top with anchovies; top with 1 layer each, roasted peppers, pepper rings and sliced tomato.

Cover with top of bread. Wrap loaf in plastic wrap. Return to plate, place in refrigerator and cover with another large plate. Put a can or other weight on top to press sandwich down.

Refrigerate 8 hours or overnight.

Unwrap and cut into 6 wedges.

Spanish Hamburgers

2 cups water
10 ounce bottle catsup
½ cup chopped onion
¼ teaspoon salt
1/8 teaspoon pepper
1/8 teaspoon red pepper
1½ teaspoons chili powder

Put all ingredients in a roasting pan and simmer 2 hours.

Fry 25 hamburgers and place burgers in roaster and refrigerate overnight.

The next day reheat and serve burgers with a little juice.

25 Servings.

Kindness is like a boomerang --
it always returns.

Spanish Burgers

2 pounds lean ground beef
1 small bunch celery
3 medium size onions
1 can (10 ounce) tomato soup
1 tablespoon worcestershire sauce
½ teaspoon salt
¼ teaspoon pepper

Brown ground beef in vegetable sprayed non stick pan.

Chop celery and onions, put over ground beef, add tomato soup and seasonings, simmer until celery is done.

18-24 Servings.

Thoughtfulness is to friendship
as sunshine is to a garden.

Asparagus Baked Sandwich

16 ounces frozen asparagus spears or fresh
1 medium onion, chopped
2 tablespoons olive oil or choice of oil
6 ounce jar sliced mushroom, drained
3 tablespoons flour
½ teaspoon seasoned salt
1/8 teaspoon pepper
½ teaspoon dried basil
1½ - 2 cups milk
4 slices grain or wheat bread, toasted

Steam asparagus according to directions on package.

Meanwhile in skillet heat the oil and sauté onions until tender. Stir in flour and seasonings, gradually stir in the milk, cook until smooth and thickened. Add the mushrooms to the sauce.

Lay toast in 10x6 inch baking dish, top with asparagus. Spoon sauce over asparagus.

Bake in 375 degrees oven 10 minutes.

4 Servings.

Mushroom Stroganoff

2 medium onions, minced
2 tablespoons olive oil
1 pound mushrooms, sliced or
        6 ounce jar sliced mushrooms, drained
2/3 cup dry red or white wine
2 tablespoons Worcestershire sauce or
        lite soy sauce
1/8 teaspoon nutmeg
1/8 teaspoon cinnamon
¼ teaspoon salt
1/8 teaspoon white pepper
2 cups fat free sour cream

In skillet heat vegetable oil, add onions and sauté until they are softened, add the mushrooms and cook, stirring for 5 minutes. Stir in the wine, Worcestershire sauce, nutmeg, cinnamon, salt and pepper to taste. Cook the mixture over medium heat until liquid is reduced some. Add the sour cream and cook until mixture is heated through, but do not let it boil. Serve the mixture over cooked rice or bread toasted.

6 Servings.

Mushroom Bordelaise Sauce
(over toast)

1 cup dry red wine
¼ cup chopped onions
1/16 teaspoon black pepper
¼ teaspoon dried thyme
½ bay leaf
10½ ounce can beef broth
¼ cup flour mixed with ½ cup water
6 ounce jar sliced mushrooms, drained
toast slices

Sauté onions in a vegetable sprayed saucepan a few minutes. Add red wine, pepper, thyme, bay leaf and beef broth. Simmer for about 10 minutes. Stir in flour mixture and continue stirring over low heat until sauce bubbles and thickens. Remove bay leaf from sauce, add mushrooms and heat a few minutes.

Serve over thin slices of toast.

4 Servings.

Laughter is the shock absorber for life's blows.

Quick Beer Wheat Bread

3 cups biscuit mix
1 cup whole wheat flour
2 tablespoons sugar
2 eggs
12 ounce can beer

In mixing bowl combine biscuit mix, flour and sugar. Add eggs and beer. Beat with electric mixer about 1 minute or until blended.

Turn into vegetable sprayed 9x5x3 inch loaf pan, spreading evenly.

Bake in 350 degrees oven for 50-60 minutes.

Cool in pan 10 minutes, Remove and cool on wire rack.

6-8 Servings.

*If we don't know what we want to do,
it's harder to do it.*

Casserole Rye Batter Bread

½ cup molasses
1 teaspoon salt
1 tablespoon butter
1½ cups very warm water
2 packages active dry yeast
2½ cups all purpose flour
2 cups unsifted rye flour

Dissolve yeast in very warm water in large bowl, mix in molasses, salt and butter, cool to luke-warm. To mixture, add the all purpose and rye flour, all at once, stir until well blended.

Cover bowl, let rise in warm place, away from draft, until double in bulk, about 50-60 minutes.

Start heating oven to 375 degrees.

Stir batter down, then beat well about 30 seconds. Turn into well sprayed, with vegetable oil, 1½ quart casserole or on well sprayed cookie sheet shaped into a round.

Bake about 40-50 minutes or until done. Turn out on wire rack to cool.

Molasses Bran Muffins

2 cups whole bran cereal
½ cup molasses
1½ cups skim milk
1 egg, beaten or egg substitute
1 cup all purpose flour
¼ teaspoon salt
1 teaspoon soda

Mix whole bran cereal with the molasses and milk. Let stand about 10 minutes. Add beaten egg to molasses mixture. Mix flour, salt and soda. Mix all ingredients together.

Fill vegetable sprayed muffin pans 2/3 full and bake in hot oven 375 degrees about 18-20 minutes.

24 – 2 inch muffins or 14 – 2 ¾ inch muffins.

14 Servings.

No Butter Stuffing

1 can (14½ ounces) chicken or turkey broth or
       1¾ cups broth
1 stalk celery, chopped
1 small onion, chopped
4 cups herb seasoned stuffing
1/16 teaspoon pepper

In medium saucepan, mix broth, pepper, celery and onion. Over high heat bring to a boil. Reduce heat to low, cover and cook 5 minutes or until vegetables are tender. Add stuffing, mix lightly.

5 Servings.

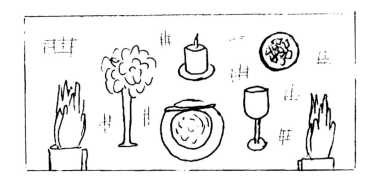

Chapter 9

Vegetables

Stir Fry Green Beans

16 ounce package French style green beans
4 ounce jar sliced mushrooms
¼ cup sliced water chestnuts, optional
½ cup broth
2 teaspoons cornstarch or arrowroot
1 tablespoon soy sauce

Steam green beans 10 minutes, add mushrooms, chestnuts and broth.

Mix cornstarch or arrowroot and soy sauce together and stir into hot vegetable. Mix well. Heat until slightly thickened.

6-8 Servings.

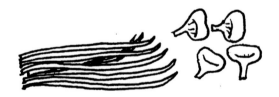

Creamed String Beans

10 ounces freezer green beans
¾ cup milk
¼ teaspoon salt
2 tablespoons flour, mixed with
        3 tablespoons water
¼ teaspoon paprika
¼ teaspoon nutmeg
3 ounces fat free cream cheese
¼ cup sliced mushrooms

Cook beans in milk according to package directions, when almost tender, add salt, flour mixture, paprika and nutmeg. Add cubed cream cheese just until melted, add mushrooms.

String Beans with Sour Cream

Cook green beans as in basic recipe, add ½ cup sour cream or yogurt in place of cream cheese.

3-4 Servings.

*Politeness is a small price to pay
for the good will and affection of others.*

Swedish Spinach

10 ounce package chopped frozen spinach
3 tablespoons flour
½ cup water
¼ teaspoon salt
1/8 teaspoon pepper
1/8 teaspoon nutmeg

Place frozen spinach in one half cup boiling water in saucepan. Bring to a second boil and add flour mixed with ½ cup water. Add salt, pepper and nutmeg.

Cover and simmer for about 10 minutes.

2-3 Servings.

*A rebuke goes deeper into a person
of understanding
than a hundred blows to a fool.*

Mashed Potatoes Casserole

32 ounce package hash brown potatoes,
   partially thawed
2 cups milk
½ teaspoon salt
2/3 cup shredded cheese, optional

Put potatoes in a vegetable oil sprayed 2 quart baking dish, separating potato pieces. Combine milk and salt, pour over potatoes. Cover with foil.

Bake in 350 degrees oven for 1¼ hours or until potatoes are fork tender. Stir half way through. Remove foil.

Can add the 2/3 cup cheese here and bake until cheese melts, about 10 minutes. Or can sprinkle lightly with paprika.

6-8 Servings.

Nothing is a waste of time
if we use the experience wisely.

Potato Beer Casserole

4 large potatoes, peeled and sliced
1 large onion, sliced
2 cups sliced celery, optional
flour
1 cup beer
1 cup chicken or turkey broth
½ teaspoon salt
1/8 teaspoon white pepper

Put layers of potato, onion and celery into a
2 quart casserole. Sprinkle small amount of flour
between potato layers.

Add beer mixed with broth, salt and pepper.
Cover and bake in 375 degrees oven for 1 hour or
until potatoes are tender.

6-8 Servings.

House and wealth are inherited from family
but a prudent spouse is from God.

Roasted Red Potatoes

1 pound small red potatoes
1 tablespoon olive oil or canola oil
½ teaspoon salt
1/8 teaspoon pepper
2 tablespoons Parmesan cheese

Cut the potatoes in ¼ inch slices, toss with oil. Place in a 13x9x2 inch baking pan. Sprinkle with salt, pepper and Parmesan cheese. Cover with foil.

Bake in 350 degrees oven for 40-45 minutes or until tender.

Take foil off, sprinkle lightly with paprika and bake 5 minutes more.

4 Servings.

Correction does much
but encouragement does more.

Cucumbers with Sour Cream

2 large cucumbers
1 cup fat free sour cream
½ teaspoon salt
1/16 teaspoon pepper
1 teaspoon dill weed
1 teaspoon chopped chives
1 tablespoon lemon juice

Peel and slice cucumbers thin; place in bowl and cover with boiling water, let stand 20 minutes, drain and put into cold water, drain and refrigerate ½ hour.

Mix sour cream with remaining ingredients, pour over cucumbers and mix.

Note: After peeling cucumbers, instead of slicing, cut cucumbers in half lengthwise, remove seeds and cut into ½ slices.

4-6 Servings.

We can always distinguish luck from ability on the basis of its duration.

Sautéed Cabbage

1 teaspoon instant bouillon
6 cups coleslaw and carrot mixture
½ cup sliced yellow onion
½ teaspoon salt
1/8 teaspoon pepper
1 teaspoon mustard
½ teaspoon dry basil, crushed
1/3 cup chopped pecans, optional

In a three quart saucepan, heat instant bouillon in 1/3 cup water until dissolved. Add onion, cabbage and carrot mixture, salt, pepper, mustard and basil, cook covered over medium heat 5-10 minutes or until tender, stirring twice during cooking. Stir in pecans if using.

Spoon into serving dish and sprinkle lightly with paprika.

4-6 Servings.

*The only sure thing about luck is
that it will change.*

Savory Beets

16 ounce can beets, sliced or diced
¼ cup sour cream
1 tablespoon tarragon or cider vinegar
½ teaspoon sugar
¼ teaspoon salt
1/16 teaspoon cayenne pepper

Heat beets, drain. While beets are heating, combine sour cream, vinegar, sugar, salt and cayenne pepper. Add to drained beets. Heat over low heat or in microwave until warmed.

4 Servings.

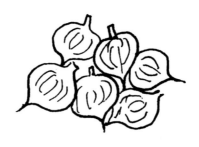

Celery Casserole

4 cups sliced celery
½ cup boiling water
10½ ounce can low fat cream of mushroom soup,
    undiluted
½ cup milk
½ cup chopped pecans

Cook celery in boiling water until tender. Drain. Combine with soup, milk and pecans; mix well. Turn into vegetable sprayed 1½ quart casserole. Sprinkle around edge with cracker crumbs if desired.

Bake in 350 degree oven for 30 minutes.

Note: Can prepare ahead of time, then bake or reheat in microwave.

6 Servings.

A face without a smile is like
a lantern without a light.

Zucchini Tomato Fans

3 sweet white onions, thinly sliced,
    separated into rings
3 cloves garlic, finely chopped
4 small firm zucchini's
3 medium tomatoes, sliced medium thin
½ teaspoon ground thyme
½ teaspoon ground oregano
¼ cup olive oil
½ cup dry white wine
½ teaspoon salt
¼ teaspoon pepper

Put half the onions and garlic in ungreased baking dish, 11¾ x 7½ x 1¾ inch. Cut zucchini in half lengthwise. Cut each half, cut side down, into lengthwise slices from wide to narrow end, keeping narrow end intact to form a fan.

Place zucchini fans, cut side down, on onion garlic mixture. Put tomato slices between slices of zucchini, spreading fans slightly. Sprinkle remaining onions and garlic on top. Mix thyme and oregano, sprinkle over onions. Drizzle olive oil over onions, repeat with wine. Sprinkle with salt and pepper. Cover baking dish.

Place in 350 degree oven. Bake until zucchini is tender but firm, about 25-35 minutes.

4-6 Servings. Serve hot or cold.

Note: If tomatoes are large, cut in half.

Braised Celery and Green Beans

6 celery stalks
10½ ounce can beef consommé, undulated
1/8 teaspoon pepper
¼ cup water
8 ounces frozen whole green beans
2 tablespoons flour dissolved in 3 Tblsp. water

Wash celery, cut off the tops and save for another use. Remove the strings. Cut each stalk into 3½ inch pieces. Cut each piece into strips about the size of green beans.

In medium saucepan, combine celery with beef consommé, pepper and ¼ cup water. Bring to boiling over medium heat, lower heat and simmer about 20-25 minutes or until celery is tender.

Meanwhile steam whole green beans according to directions on package.

Remove celery from saucepan and arrange in stacks with green beans alternately on serving dish

Thicken liquid in saucepan with the flour and water mixture. Spoon the sauce over celery and beans. Sprinkle with chopped parsley if desired.

4-6 Servings.

Note: Spooning thickened sauce over celery and beans is optional. Sprinkle only with chopped parsley if desired.

Golden Carrots

2 cups frozen sliced carrots, thawed
20½ ounce can unsweetened pineapple chunks
1/8 teaspoon nutmeg
1½ tablespoons cornstarch or arrowroot

Steam carrots about 10 minutes. Put carrots in saucepan along with the pineapple chunks, including juice and nutmeg. Bring to a boil add the cornstarch dissolved in 2 tablespoons water. Heat, stirring until thickened. Serve.

6 Servings.

Note: Can cut pineapple chunks in half, if desired.

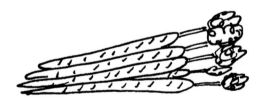

Broccoli Dish

10 ounce package frozen broccoli spears,
    thawed and well drained
4 eggs, lightly beaten or egg beaters
½ teaspoon salt
½ teaspoon nutmeg
1¼ cups milk
½ cup grated mozzarella cheese

Preheat oven to 350 degrees.

Mix eggs with salt and nutmeg. Add milk and cheese, beating constantly. Pour into oil sprayed shallow baking dish, 9 inch pie plate is good. Add broccoli spears, that have been separated, large ones cut in half lengthwise and pressed with a paper towel to get moisture out of the spears, arrange in a spoke like circle.

Bake 40 – 50 minutes or until knife inserted in center comes out clean.

4-5 Servings.

Sautéed Onions

2 tablespoons water
1 teaspoon oil
1/2 cup sliced or chopped onions

Place in a small saucepan the water, the oil and the onions.
Simmer, covered, 5 minutes. Uncover and brown the onions.

1 serving.

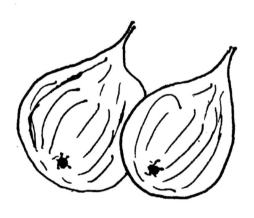

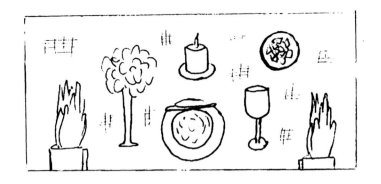

Chapter 10

Desserts

Hot Fruit Compote

1 cup prunes
8 ounce can pineapple chunks, drained
1 cup frozen peaches, sliced
1 cup dried apricots
2 cups unsweetened applesauce
1 teaspoon cinnamon
½ teaspoon ginger
½ teaspoon nutmeg
Juice of ½ lemon & its rind grated

Mix seasonings in the applesauce and fold in the fruits, place in a covered casserole dish in a 250-275 degree oven for at lease 1 hour before serving.

Serve hot or cold.

6-8 Servings.

*Pray for a good harvest,
but continue to hoe.*

Steamed Cranberry Pudding

½ cup molasses
2 teaspoons baking soda in ½ cup hot water
1 1/3 cups flour
½ - 1 cup nuts, chopped
1½ cups cranberries, each sliced in half

Mix all ingredients together in a large bowl. Place the mixture in a greased mold on a trivet over water in a kettle, cover mold with wax paper, cover kettle & steam it for about 2 hours.

6-8 Servings.

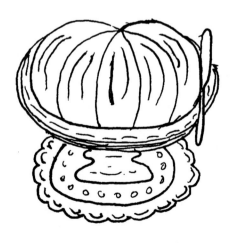

Rice Pudding

2 cups skim milk
½ cup egg beaters
¼ cup sugar
1 tablespoon cornstarch or arrowroot
2 teaspoons vanilla
2 cups cooked rice
ground nutmeg

Heat milk in saucepan until very warm.

Mix egg beaters, sugar, cornstarch and vanilla. Gradually stir into milk. Heat and stir until it comes to a boil and boils 1 minute. Stir in rice. Put in bowl, cover with plastic wrap and chill 3 hours.

When serving sprinkle lightly with nutmeg.

4 Servings.

Luck is where preparation meets opportunity.

Pumpkin Pudding

15 ounce can plain pumpkin
3 ounce package instant vanilla pudding,
can be sugar free
1 cup milk
2 teaspoons pumpkin pie spice

Beat all ingredients together until smooth. Chill
in serving bowl or individual dessert dishes.

4 Servings.

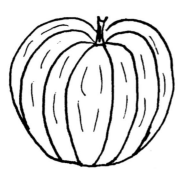
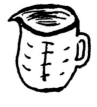

Pineapple Sherbet

20 ounce can unsweetened pineapple chunks,
that has been frozen and slightly thawed.

Puree the slightly thawed chunks in a blender or food processor until smooth, thick and creamy, about 2 minutes.

Note: Can refreeze some of the puree in serving size.

4 Servings.

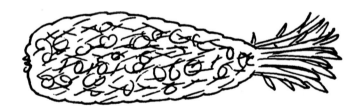

Quick Fruit Salad or Dessert

6 canned pineapple slices
6 canned peach halves
6 canned whole apricots
2 cups fat free yogurt, plain or flavored
Salad greens

Chill and drain fruits thoroughly.

Place a lettuce leaf on serving dish. Top with pineapple slice, put on spoonful yogurt, sprinkle with cinnamon or nutmeg. Place peach half, cut side up, over yogurt, fill center of peach with yogurt, sprinkle lightly with cinnamon or nutmeg. Top with apricot.

6 Servings.

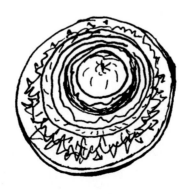

Dessert Pancakes

1 cup all purpose flour
1/16 teaspoon salt
1/16 teaspoon nutmeg
1 egg
1½ cups fat free milk
all fruit type jam or preserves

Blend dry ingredients; add egg and milk, beat thoroughly with electric mixer or rotary beater.

Using a ¼ cup measure, not full, pour on vegetable oil sprayed heated griddle or skillet. Lightly brown on one side, turn over and lightly brown on the other side.

Spread each cake with all fruit type jam or preserves, roll up. Sprinkle lightly with confectioners sugar.

Makes about ten 5" pancakes.

Each time you turn the pages
Looking for something new to cook
Fondly remember the person
Who made possible this book.

Fruit Pumpkin Bake

16 ounce can pumpkin
1 1/3 cups nonfat dry milk
½ teaspoon pumpkin pie spice
¼ teaspoon vanilla
2 cups unsweetened applesauce

Combine all ingredients. Put mixture in shallow baking dish, lightly sprayed with vegetable oil.

Bake in 350 degrees oven for 50 – 60 minutes.

Serve warm or chilled with a dollop of fat free whipped topping or yogurt sprinkled lightly with cinnamon.

5 Servings.

*Tact is the ability to close your mouth
before someone else wants to.*

Chocolate Cheesecake

½ cup chocolate cookie crumbs
4 eight ounce packages fat free cream cheese,
    softened
16 ounce container ready to spread
    chocolate frosting
4 large eggs
strawberries for garnish, optional

Spray well a 9 x 3 inch spring form pan, cover bottom of pan with the chocolate cookie crumbs.

In large bowl, with mixer at medium speed, beat cream cheese and chocolate frosting until smooth, scraping bowl often with rubber spatula. Add eggs; beat just until blended. Pour cream cheese mixture over crumbs in pan.

Bake cheesecake 1 hour in a 350 degree oven.

Cool cheesecake in pan on wire rack.

Refrigerate cheesecake at least 6 hours.

To serve, carefully remove side of springform pan. Place cheesecake on a cake plate.

Garnish each serving with chocolate drizzle and a strawberry if desired.

18-20 Servings.

Note: Can prepare a day ahead.

Strawberries with Balsamic Vinegar

1 pint strawberries, washed and hulled
2 teaspoons balsamic vinegar
Freshly ground pepper

Just before serving, toss strawberries, in a bowl, with vinegar and pepper.

4 Servings.

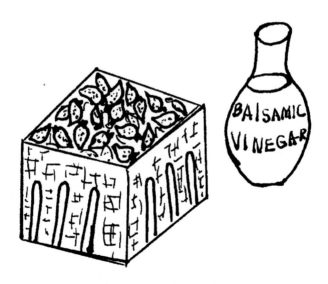

Fat – Free Cheesecake

1 tablespoon Graham cracker crumbs
1 ½ cups nonfat cottage cheese
1 cup egg substitute
½ cup sugar
½ cup nonfat cream cheese
1 tablespoon lemon juice
¼ teaspoon grated lemon peel

Spray bottom and sides of spring form pan with cooking spray. Sprinkle graham cracker crumbs over bottom and about ½ inch up side. Set aside.

In electric blender or food processor, blend cottage cheese and ½ cup egg substitute until smooth. Combine with remaining egg substitute, sugar, cream cheese, lemon juice and peel. Beat at low speed 2 minutes.

Pour into prepared pan. Bake at 325 degrees oven for 50 minutes or until set and lightly browned. Cool in pan on wire rack. Chill 2 hours.

9 Servings.

Oatmeal Applesauce Cookies

1 cup dates
¾ cup oil
1 cup applesauce
1 teaspoon vanilla
½ cup chopped nuts
½ teaspoon salt
4 cups oatmeal
½ cup chopped raisins, optional

Blend oil and dates together in blender. Add to applesauce and vanilla mixed. Stir in remaining ingredients and mix well.

Drop by teaspoons onto cookie sheets, which has been lined with foil and sprayed with vegetable oil. Flatten cookies slightly.

Bake in 325 degrees oven for 20-25 minutes or until lightly browned.

Let cool before removing from pan.

Makes 5-6 dozen cookies. - 2 cookies per serving.

One Bowl Bar Cookie

1 package applesauce - raisin cake mix
¾ cup oatmeal
¼ cup wheat germ
½ cup light molasses
¼ cup pineapple juice
2 eggs
2 tablespoons vegetable oil
½ cup raisins

Combine cake mix, oats and wheat germ. Add molasses, pineapple juice, eggs and oil; stir until well blended. Stir in raisins.

Spread in vegetable sprayed 15x10x1 inch jelly roll pan. Bake in 375 degree oven about 20 minutes or until cookies are lightly browned and pull away from edge of pan. Cool.

Cut into 1½ x 2 inch bars. Sprinkle lightly with confectioners sugar if desired.

25 Servings.

Crustless Pumpkin Pie

15 ounce can plain pumpkin
12 ounce can evaporated skim milk
2 eggs substitute
2 egg whites
¾ cup sugar
1 teaspoon cinnamon
½ teaspoon ginger
1/8 teaspoon salt
½ cup graham cracker crumbs

In mixing bowl, combine the pumpkin, milk, egg substitute, egg whites and sugar, beat until smooth. Add the spices and salt, beat until well mixed. Stir in graham cracker crumbs. Pour into 9 inch pie plate coated with non-stick cooking spray.

Bake in 325 degrees oven for 50-55 minutes or until knife inserted in center comes out clean. Cool.

8 Servings.

Cranberry - Apple Walnut Pie

Pastry for a 9 inch 2 crust pie

4 cups, pared apples, sliced
2 cups, fresh or frozen, cranberries
1 cup walnuts, chopped
½ cup brown sugar
¼ cup sugar
3 tablespoons flour
1 teaspoon cinnamon

Preheat oven to 425 degrees.

In large bowl combine brown sugar, sugar, flour and cinnamon. Stir in apples, cranberries and walnuts, combine thoroughly. Pour filling into pastry lined pie plate.

Cover with top crust. Seal and flute edges, make several slits in top crust.

Bake 50 minutes.

8 Servings.

Crustless Persian Pie

1 dozen dates, chopped
½ cup pecans, chopped
½ - ¾ cup sugar
1 dozen soda crackers, crushed fine
½ teaspoon baking powder
1 teaspoon vanilla extract
3 large egg whites, stiffly beaten

Mix first five ingredients. Fold in vanilla and stiffly beaten egg whites.

Pour into an 8 or 9 inches pie pan, which has been well sprayed with vegetable oil.

Bake in 350 degrees oven for 30 minutes.

Let cool before cutting.

6-8 Servings.

It's a little too much to save
And a little too much to dump
And there's nothing to do but eat it
That makes this body plump!

Frozen Pumpkin Squares

7 whole graham crackers
½ gallon soft vanilla fat free and
      sugar free frozen yogurt
15 ounce can plain pumpkin
1 teaspoon ginger
½ teaspoon nutmeg
1 teaspoon cinnamon

Line 13x9x2 inch pan with crackers.

Combine remaining ingredients, pour mixture over crackers. Cover with foil and freeze overnight or about 4 hours.

Can sprinkle top with graham cracker crumbs.

Cut into 12 or more squares.

12 Servings.

Looking for the best in others
brings out the best in us.

Pie Crust (Double Crust)

½ cup salad oil
¼ cup milk
1 teaspoon salt
2 cups flour

Mix flour and salt in mixing bowl, mix salad oil and milk, add to flour mixture, stir until mixed. Divide dough in half. Put one half between 2 sheets of waxed paper (12 inch square), flatten slightly. Roll out to edge of paper. Peel off top paper. Place paper side up in 8- or 9-inch pie plate. Peel off paper, ease and fit pastry into pan.

Top Crust
Roll as above and place over filling. Fold edges under bottom crust. Seal by pressing with fork over edge, trim or by fluting edge. Cut slits in crust for steam to escape.

For Single Pie Crust
Mix flour and salt in pie plate. Mix milk and oil and pour over flour mixture. Mix with fork until mixed. Press evenly and firmly with fingers to line bottom of pan, then press dough up to line sides and rim. Be sure dough is pressed to uniform thickness. Press edge with fork or lightly flute edge.

Easy Peanut Butter Cookies

1 package yellow cake mix
1 cup crunchy peanut butter
½ cup vegetable oil
2 tablespoons water
2 eggs

Combine all ingredients and mix well. Drop from a teaspoon onto an ungreased cookie sheet, flatten with a fork.

Bake in a preheated 350 degree oven for 10 – 12 minutes.

Yield: 5 dozen cookies.

Note: Can substitute 1 package chocolate cake mix for some delicious chocolate cookies.

Chocolate – Nut Fruit Balls

8 ounce package pitted dates, chopped
1¼ cups dark raisins, chopped
1 cup pitted prunes, chopped
1 cup chopped pecans
½ cup semi-sweet chocolate mini morsels
2 tablespoons rum
finely chopped pecans

Combine fruits, 1 cup pecans, the chocolate and rum. Shape ½ tablespoon of the fruit mixture into a ball, roll in finely chopped pecans or drop ½ tablespoon of the fruit mixture into the finely chopped nuts and shape into a ball.

Place in bonbon paper and put in a cookie canister. Refrigerate, covered, overnight.

Makes about 4 dozen.

Note: I coarsely chopped the fruits, separately, in a food processor.

Also chopped semi – sweet chocolate morsels can be substituted for the mini morsels.

THINK
THIN

RECIPE INDEX